THE CREATIVE THERAPIST IN PRACTICE

In *The Creative Therapist in Practice* Hillary and Bradford Keeney present a radically innovative approach to the practice of therapy. Combining improvisational performing arts, action-oriented cybernetics, and ecstatic healing traditions, therapy is re-imagined as a creative transformative art.

The book demonstrates the principles of creative therapy through numerous transcriptions of sessions conducted by the authors. It guides practitioners in conducting a three-part therapeutic performance: beginning with therapeutic techniques that broaden the context, igniting a session to creatively "cook," and finally concluding with a creative prescription for change that can be incorporated into the client's daily living. As well as tracing the historical development of creative therapy, chapters explore what is possible for the future of therapy when practitioners leave behind conventional models and theoretical interpretations.

Applying case examples of creative therapy to a wide range of presenting concerns, *The Creative Therapist in Practice* will be relevant to clinicians working across the field of mental health, including licensed psychotherapists, psychologists, and clinical social workers. Filled with inspiring anecdotes, unique interventions, and fascinating case illustrations, it will benefit anyone looking to become more naturally improvisational and wake up the creative life force in their sessions.

Hillary Keeney, PhD, is Director, Institute for Creative Therapy, Distinguished Visiting Professor at Benemérita Universidad Autónoma de Puebla, and Associate Editor of the journal, *Dance, Movement, and Spiritualities*.

Bradford Keeney, PhD, is the former director of several clinical doctoral programs, an improvisational pianist, and an explorer of creative approaches to psychotherapy.

"This book brought me great surprise and delight as the Keeneys, the audacious creative therapists of our time, tread where most therapists fear to go. Their innovative interventions seem magical, but are here clearly shown as inspired by novel ideas and powerful techniques that activate change. This book will truly inspire and challenge you to change how you perform and reform your practice."

PEGGY PAPP, LCSW, a founder of family therapy and faculty, Ackerman Institute for the Family

"Goethe wrote: 'All theory, dear friend, is gray; but the golden tree of life springs ever green.' Hillary and Brad offer 'the wake-up zap, the exuberant tap, and the rhyming rap' to add zing and swing to make your sessions sing. Inspired by Carl Whitaker, Milton Erickson, and Gregory Bateson, as well as improvisational performance and healing traditions around the world, *The Creative Therapist in Practice* invites clinicians and their clients into greater aliveness, hope, love, healing and health. Roll over, Beethoven, the Keeneys are in the house!"

MICHAEL F. HOYT, PhD, Author/editor, *Brief Therapy and Beyond*, *Therapist Stories of Inspiration, Passion, and Renewal*, and *Single-Session Therapy by Walk-In or Appointment*

"The Keeneys have created a beautiful and magical book. Its graceful blend of imagination and wisdom brings a creative therapeutic performance that goes far beyond interpretation. Watch out, this rich counter–therapy–culture message with its long-lasting effect deserves widespread attention!"

DAVID KEITH, MD, Professor of Psychiatry and Family Medicine, Director of Family Therapy, SUNY Upstate Medical University, and author of *Continuing the Experiential Approach of Carl Whitaker: Process, Practice, and Magic*

"I don't know how to adequately convey that the Keeneys are true to the work of Milton H. Erickson."

BETTY ALICE ERICKSON, MS, International teacher of psychotherapy

"A thirst-quenching revitalization of the experiential approach to eliciting change that is based on evocative orientations, arousal states, and artistic improvisation. The Keeneys' innovations turn the parched earth of academic psychotherapy into an oasis for both the client and the clinician."

JEFFREY K. ZEIG, PhD, The Milton H. Erickson Foundation

"The Keeneys have the gift of helping people change. As authentic healers with impeccable scholarship, they bring us inside the heart of transformation and the soul of exuberant, creative living."

PAUL TRACHTMAN, Former Science Editor, *Smithsonian Magazine*

"Creative therapy brings the excitement and surprise found in the improvised performance of theatre, poetry, dance, and music. This is not a theory; it is a radical call for the kind of *experience* that changes lives. Move over, Shiva, the Keeneys are recreating therapy!"

STEPHEN LANKTON, LCSW, DAHB, FASCH, Editor-in-Chief, *American Journal of Clinical Hypnosis* and author, *The Answer Within* and *Tools of Intention*

THE CREATIVE THERAPIST IN PRACTICE

Hillary Keeney and Bradford Keeney

Routledge
Taylor & Francis Group
NEW YORK AND LONDON

First published 2019
by Routledge
52 Vanderbilt Avenue, New York, NY 10017

and by Routledge
2 Park Square, Milton Park, Abingdon, Oxon, OX14 4RN

Routledge is an imprint of the Taylor & Francis Group, an informa business

Library of Congress Cataloging-in-Publication Data
A catalog record for this title has been requested

ISBN: 978-0-367-07807-2 (hbk)
ISBN: 978-0-367-07808-9 (pbk)
ISBN: 978-0-429-02290-6 (ebk)

Typeset in Minion
by Deanta Global Publishing Services, Chennai, India

This book is dedicated to our dear friend and colleague,
Dezsoe Birkas, MD

CONTENTS

PART I
The Basics

1

THE HISTORICAL DEVELOPMENT OF CREATIVE THERAPY

The seeds for creative therapy were planted in the early 1970s. At that time, Brad was an improvisational pianist and social cybernetician already steeped in the ideas of Gregory Bateson and Heinz von Foerster. He had little interest in psychotherapy and used to joke that he found the therapy profession more in need of therapy than its clients. As a young teacher of undergraduate psychology whose main academic interest was sensory-perception neurobiology, Brad conducted an unusual experiment. The students were shown a classic film series of sessions conducted by various founders of psychotherapy, but told that some of them were schizophrenics pretending to be therapists. After viewing the tapes, Brad asked the students to point out who the real therapists were. He was shocked to discover that the undergraduate students—not yet indoctrinated in psychological discourse—diagnosed most of the famous therapists as crazy imposters. This outcome made a long-lasting impression on Brad's skeptical view of what is accepted and taught as therapeutic performance.

Then Brad attended a workshop conducted by Carl Whitaker in the spring of 1975 that was hosted by the institute where Brad worked as a researcher. Whitaker conducted a live interview with a family in front of the audience and it struck Brad as more an example of incredibly inspiring theater than any kind of therapy. What took place on stage appeared as a unique genre of improvisational performance—its transformative power was palpable. There was no need to assess, rationalize, or persuade anyone that a therapeutic outcome had taken place—it was immediately and obviously experienced by everyone in the room.

Afterwards Brad introduced himself to Carl Whitaker and the two of them started an immediate friendship that lasted through Brad's early academic career. Whitaker asked Brad what he witnessed in the session and Brad responded without mentioning a single psychological abstraction or theoretical hypothesis. His words were limited to the patterns observed and the experiences evoked. Whitaker, known as a maverick practitioner who distrusted models and theories, immediately invited Brad to enter the field of psychotherapy and bring this kind of non-theoretical, performance-oriented, and cybernetic pattern-attuned perspective to the profession. When Brad asked Whitaker how he learned to perform in a therapeutic session, he was little prepared for his answer. Whitaker replied, "I am fortunate because I was never trained. I did not have to unlearn those habits that bring the kiss of death to a session. I learned how to follow my unconscious instincts, chasing whatever wakes up a session and makes it feel alive. I am a non-theoretical, experiential family therapist." Brad followed Whitaker's advice and eschewed all training. Even while pursuing a doctorate in family therapy, he managed to avoid clinical supervision, instead getting faculty approval to set up an experimental project on a new method of therapy he invented, insinuating it was being studied at the Menninger Foundation where he worked as a communications analyst. Like Whitaker, Brad remained an untrained therapist, that is, uninfluenced by conventional schools of therapy.

Hillary began her career with much the same skepticism regarding psychotherapy that Brad had as a young man. Her interdisciplinary scholarship focused on social justice movements, Zen Buddhism, and dance. Then one day Hillary witnessed Brad conduct a live session with a married couple in front of an audience. The performance was so transformative and moving the audience laughed, wept, and erupted in applause. She had no idea that psychotherapy could be this creative, theatrical, and electric. Hillary refocused her scholarship on cybernetics as a tool for discerning how a therapy session is constructed by performed interaction rather than construed by informed interpretation. Performance oriented with aesthetic sensitivity and cybernetic pragmatic chops, Hillary partnered with Brad in the development and elaboration of what today is called creative therapy.

Creative therapy was able to sprout and grow only after the ground was swept clear of unnecessary explanatory principles—especially of the psychological and psychiatric kind. Rather than house therapy in social science or medicine, from the very beginning it was situated in the performing arts, having kinship with the kind of thrilling performance Brad initially witnessed by Whitaker and further developed in his own clinical work. Creative therapy's developmental journey is radically free of psychology's influence, but therapeutically enriched by several other lineages. These include theatrically setting a stage and making an enacted drama of transformation come to life. Add to this a few practical ideas from cybernetics that emphasize circular interaction and the co-construction of realities, and practitioners are better equipped to improvise rather than recycle a memorized routine.

Next widen the range of expression that is possible in a session, something better acquired from other arenas of performance that include theater, dance, and music. And finally, become tutored by numerous global healing traditions that never forgot that change is something more felt than understood, and is best served when a practitioner is plugged into the ineffable source of the creative life force. Mix all this together and you have the creative therapist in practice—an innovative approach to therapy that uniquely blends the know-how of the performing arts, the wisdom of traditional healing ways, and the systemic understanding provided by the cybernetics of therapeutic interaction.

The Beginning: Exploring the Cybernetics of Change

The seminal ideas behind our unique therapeutic approach came into publication in the early days of Brad's career when he served as Director of Research at the Ackerman Institute for Family Therapy in New York City and later as the director of several doctoral graduate programs. His first published book, *Aesthetics of Change* (Keeney, 1983), used the basic concepts of cybernetics, especially those articulated by Gregory Bateson, Heinz von Foerster, and Francisco Varela, to describe therapeutic change. Heinz von Foerster, one of the founders of cybernetics, cited *Aesthetics of Change* as a key general textbook on cybernetics in his entry on "cybernetics" in the *Encyclopedia of Artificial Intelligence*. Whereas Gregory Bateson earlier presented the ideas of Norbert Wiener to the social sciences, Brad gave more contextual clarification of the historical definition of these ideas, introduced their relationship to later developments of second-order cybernetics, and suggested how cybernetic metaphor could both describe and prescribe therapeutic process.

His next published books, *Mind in Therapy* (Keeney & Ross, 1985) and *The Therapeutic Voice of Olga Silverstein* (Keeney & Silverstein, 1986), used this cybernetic perspective to discern relevant patterns of communication in the sessions of renowned therapists that included Olga Silverstein, John Weakland, Jay Haley, Salvador Minuchin, H. Charles Fishman, Luigi Boscolo, and Gianfranco Cecchin. He demonstrated how therapeutic change could be discerned with a few primary distinctions, helping prevent any unnecessary multiplication of explanatory principles that dissociate attention away from the actual performance. His emerging orientation of scholarship combined cybernetic epistemology with a specific means of distinguishing the primary distinctions upon which any kind of experienced reality is built, a method inspired by George Spencer Brown's *Laws of Form* (1969), a seminal contribution to logic and mathematics. As a "radical constructivist," as it was called back then, Brad depicted a client and therapist as co-constructing a session's reality through the primary metaphors they cast and wove together via their circular interaction.

Moving Therapy to the Performing Arts

Later, as Director of a clinical doctoral program at Texas Tech University, Brad turned his descriptive method of analysis upside down and used it as a prescriptive strategy to invent new forms of therapy. In this phase of his career, he originated several approaches to therapy that encouraged improvisation rather than model replication, that is, the creative invention of a unique therapeutic reality for each session and client, something he also found exemplified in the work of Milton H. Erickson. Variously called "cybernetic brief therapy," "improvisational therapy," "resource focused therapy," and finally, "creative therapy," Brad began building an archive of transcribed sessions that demonstrate an orientation not bound by a singular therapeutic model, but one that is a creative means of inventing endless therapies in real time with diverse clients.

During this time, Brad wrote a book called *Improvisational Therapy* (1991) that was arguably the first treatise calling for a postmodern second-order cybernetic orientation— a "therapy of therapy." Heralded by postmodern anthropologist Professor Stephen Tyler, Brad's work exemplified therapeutic experimentalism, improvisation, and an authentic liberation from attachment to either a preferred interpretation or interpretation itself, instead favoring expressive performance less constrained, filtered, and colored by theoretical allegiance. In other words, this work sought a performance (like Carl Whitaker) that truly embodied the postmodern sentiment that frees one from advocating for or imposing any ideology, including postmodernism, instead inspired by the unique particularities of action and understanding evoked by the situation at hand (like Milton Erickson). The first sentence of *Improvisational Therapy* (Keeney, 1991, p. 1), written nearly three decades ago, announced this radical move out of the clinic and onto the performance stage: "Imagine psychotherapy being contextualized in an academy of performing arts as a discipline comfortably related to theater, music, dance, and the rhetorical arts."

This shift in context brought an emphasis on the performance of change with no need for exalting interpretation, whether it was named psychodynamic, behavioral, interactional, cybernetic, or postmodern, something unimaginable to a profession that typically believes its universe is a battlefield of contested interpretations and evangelical-like advocacy for a preferred ideology, even when the latter is an ideology concerning the deconstruction of other ideologies.

Brad found that opposition to one side of a polarity often results in an unnoticed conversion to what is opposed, what the Greeks (and later Carl Jung) named "enantiodromia." Or as we now often humorously say, "too much protest leads to the love nest." Opponents of traditional psychological interpretation fell into the same epistemological trap where "viewing" was elevated over "doing." For instance, the very name adopted by Watzlawick and his Mental Research Institute (MRI) colleagues for their approach, "the interactional view" (an orientation we value) shows they did not detect their own pragmatic blind spot—they did not see that they did not see that a change of view is only more of the same kind of change—one that promotes the primacy of viewing. In other words, a change of outlook or perspective alone does not necessarily facilitate interactions that promote change. Here the more you try to advance the *idea* of interaction, the more you might be led to interpreting interaction and promoting an interactional ideology and its self-verifying reality.

More significantly, schools of therapy missed underscoring that change should involve more than the client—the therapist and the model of change must also be ready to change in each session. If a client and therapist are in a circular interaction together, then they will either change together or remain the same together. While the MRI model of change came closer than other models to identifying the importance of circular interaction, they did not fully apply it or embody it in their own involvement—MRI sessions and their therapists remained predictably the same. This model only addressed one kind of interaction—the interaction of problems and attempted solutions—while ignoring whatever or whoever else is included in an interaction with a client (unless involved in solution attempts). Until the whole therapist is interacting with the whole client, there is a dissociated situation in which only parts of the therapist and parts of the client are invited to the session as determined by the therapy model. Here is found the main form of interaction implicit in all therapy models: a therapist's theoretical model is what interacts with the client, while the rest of the therapist remains constrained or removed from the situation. Carl Whitaker intuited this systemic partiality of a theoretically driven therapist. He was the only therapist to protest "the hindrance of theory" in clinical work (Whitaker, 1976). Though he wasn't sure how to best articulate or rationalize it, he invited therapists to jump into the whole system of interaction that invites more forms of participation, especially those involving their more unconscious and unpredictable creative nature.

Without such participatory inclusion and performance plasticity, a model and its practitioners are rendered change resistant in order to maintain a particular viewpoint. The art of change requires the doing and viewing that embrace an ever-shifting approach to improvising transformation. In other words, the method, school, and orientation of change must itself be changing along with its proponents, which is something not easy to understand, enact, or teach.

Brad avoided promoting a non-changing model of change that was impervious to a self-corrective process that could alter its own protocol. He noticed early on how the main therapy models implicitly sought to prioritize verification of their own utopian outlook and unavoidably stumbled into the same theoretical entrapment, myopic preferentialism, and political evangelism seen in the works and institutions they critiqued. Brad chose to explore how an emphasis on freshly invented performance rather than an imposed, stale template would better serve transformation. He also learned that saying less about either cybernetics or a postmodern sentiment could better evoke, embody, sustain, and grow both. He kept changing his metaphors and even the name of his therapy to help keep it more creatively alive and more resistant to becoming change resistant.

Scoring Therapy's Performance

Brad next invented a breakthrough research method that enabled an investigator to track and score the construction of a transformative conversation in any context concerned with the evocation of change. Later completed with Hillary, this method is called "Recursive Frame Analysis" (RFA). It reveals the barebones structure or conversational anatomy of what is going on (and what is not going on) in a therapy session no matter its theoretical orientation. Its analysis outlines the contextual frames that a therapist and client knowingly or unknowingly establish in their interaction. It makes clear whether or not an alternative experiential reality has been constructed or whether the therapist remains inside the same presenting context of the client or another equivalent analog of it. RFA tracks how the contextual space needed for a creative therapy session is built by highlighting an engaging, resourceful metaphor that, through successive re-indication and effective conversational weaving, becomes an expanded frame or existential "room" hosting a wider spectrum of transformative experience (Keeney, Keeney, & Chenail, 2015).

This innovative mapping also brought a tool for constructing new territory. RFA is equivalent to scoring music or notating the choreography of dance—a simultaneous description of and prescription for a performance. Imagine music and dance without their means of scoring—the absence of such a map would leave performers lost and students would find it nearly impossible to learn how to perform and compose. This actually has been the situation in psychotherapy—it has lacked the kind of map, score, and notational system that is performance oriented. Instead, it advances interpretations that are of a different level of abstraction, making more opaque what is happening in a session and more difficult to discern whether a session moves from a beginning, then to a middle, and finally to a transformed ending. As a result, the actual performance is often minimized or ignored altogether in favor of hosting debates on what therapists should think and how they should view rather than examining what they actually do.

Though not reported, RFA clearly revealed that most models and schools of therapy rarely achieve any significant contextual expansion nor any powerful *experience* of change in the session—echoing what Brad's undergraduates had intuited in their untrained observations of therapy films. Proponents of mainstream therapy models are usually more concerned with rationalizing and fantasizing that change occurs in their sessions even when it is not immediately perceived. Like a performing arts academy, most of the educational curriculum and conferences in psychotherapy *should* involve live session performance, something Brad required in his graduate programs and presentations over the years. The stage should be the main focus, not theoretical reflection and speculation. Furthermore, a performance and not a multiple-choice exam better determines whether a student is ready to see clients. Without the primacy of auditions, recitals, and master performance classes, therapy too easily falls into action paralysis and performance amnesia. Therapy needs less abstract theoretical fantasy and more live performance—something that naturally occurs when it is resituated in the performing arts.

Early in his career, Brad heard Gregory Bateson declare that psychotherapy was more schizophrenic than anyone dare recognize. When Brad later shared this idea with Whitaker, he heard a typically Whitakeresque response: "Everyone is crazy. The better question is asking whether you are going to get paid for it or locked up for it." Whitaker reminded him of a family therapy conference on schizophrenia that had occurred at the Barbizon Plaza Hotel in New York City. In the middle of the proceedings Jay Haley stood and protested that no human being was schizophrenic; it was, as Bateson and his team had shown, more a pattern of communication that served social adaptation than it was an individual's mental disease. All eyes at the conference then turned to Whitaker to hear what he might say since he was widely regarded for his brilliant work with so-called schizophrenics. Whitaker responded, "I've actually never met anyone who wasn't schizophrenic." It takes some circular thinking to recognize that Haley and Whitaker were saying the same thing in two different ways. However, the difference that Whitaker's connotation brings is the further implication that the client and the therapist are not that different. Something bigger must be enacted than simply proving who is the therapist and who is the client, as Bateson once described the basic nature of therapeutic interaction. Escaping the ideology of therapy models that maintain their view more than transform a situation requires the kind of interaction that can change all participants. To find this expanded range of experience, Brad turned to the global healing traditions where healers already knew that they must change themselves in order to help change another person.

Fieldwork with Global Healing Traditions

In the middle of his career, Brad took a sabbatical to conduct fieldwork with healers from indigenous cultures throughout the world. This work lasted over a decade and resulted in numerous books on diverse healing ways (Keeney, 1999–2004). This opportunity enabled him to apply what he had done in the performance analysis of therapy to that of healing practice, discerning how healing realities are constructed, maintained, and altered. Brad became immersed and formally initiated in diverse healing traditions as well as an active member of their communities. Over the years his investigations of healing involved him as both a seasoned participant and a maverick scholar.

In his fieldwork, other cultures' healing practices, epistemologies, and realities (their own metaphors, treatment methods, ways of knowing, and preferred forms of expression) were respected rather than fit into a western model of anthropology or therapy. Brad regarded these cultures as having different recipes for constructing realities that do not need to be filtered through the lens of an anthropologist or therapist whose ideology precedes their involvement. RFA enabled the healers' own means of construction to be highlighted rather than reinterpreted and reframed. This approach is different than when a white person teaches members of another culture how to be political, theoretical, or therapeutic via means that differ from their traditional ways. Brad instead advocated that healing contexts that are different from the world of therapy be accepted on equal terms. Rather than aim to produce a Maori narrative therapist, a Lakota solution-focused therapist, a Guarani cognitive therapist, or a Zulu psychoanalyst, it is far more respectful and less colonizing to allow them to bring their own linguistic terms and styles of healing to the mental health clinic, or to keep them out of the clinic if they so choose. Then we honor the differences and all our relations rather than teach others to accept the epistemology and practices of conventional therapies.

The main difference between so-called traditional healing and modern folk healing traditions, (which is how we regard psychotherapy, body therapy, and other contemporary approaches) was found in the space that hosts the performance. Traditional healing ceremonies assure that the performance context is *existentially vast* before commencing any therapeutic action. In addition, strong emotion is evoked that brings a sense of wonder and mystery. Nothing about the performance seems "clinical," but is a well-executed aesthetic production. Brad also found that "ecstatic" healing ways never regard "talk" as the "cure." If anything, talk and thought are assumed to be the source of or a contributing factor in the distress. When he described therapy to the Kalahari Bushman (San) healers, they thought he was teasing them. When he role-played a typical therapy session, they fell to the ground convulsing with laughter. Afterwards they said, "Those doctors are in need of healing."

In cultures with well-established ecstatic healing traditions, there is no such thing as minimizing or banning heightened emotion and its expression from the treatment of suffering. What takes place is more comparable to the spontaneous combustion of religious fervor than the talk found in a clinical office. Unless a session emotionally and passionately comes to life, it is believed that healing hasn't kicked into motion. The emotional excitement of ecstatic healing is somewhat comparable to Carl Whitaker's quest to *feel alive* in therapy, the experience he prioritized in a session. Brad found Whitaker's work provided a bridge from therapy to ecstatic healing: a session can't start cooking until the room feels energetically alive.

When examined through RFA we see that an ecstatic healing ceremony first builds enough existential room to host its wide range of experience. Here a sacred metaphor, symbol, or context marker is introduced and then continuously re-emphasized. This construction of ceremonial space may include ritual cleansing of the room, incense, prayer, chant, percussion, and song. When the context, space, or room is vast enough, an energized emotion (often regarded by healers as a "life force" or "spiritual energy") suddenly feels present. This is the transitional moment when the former reality seems left behind as healing ground is experientially entered. Excitement circulates among all the participants as healing has now begun and change is in the air. Only when the room becomes big enough to *feel* that the room has changed, do people experience transformation in operation.

This existential expansion is the first key to understanding how a creative therapist, like a healer, helps create a situation that is conducive to change. As Milton Erickson described it, "a favorable climate" must be created within which the client is more able to learn, change, and transform. As will be further elaborated in the next chapter, this is the first step of creative therapy in practice. What we call a "big room" must be built before *experienced change* (rather than hypothesized change) is possible. Without a big room, a session cannot go anywhere transformative, the unfortunate plight and non-flight of too many therapies. While master healers and therapists expand the room tacitly, the method of RFA enables this construction to be explicitly outlined, revealing the actual architecture of a session's contextual structure, the existential room in which it experientially rather than theoretically takes place.

An outside observer who reduces helping and change-oriented conduct to a theoretically preferred and extracted part, factor, or element is vulnerable to missing what else is occurring in the immediate phenomenal field. The entire room of a session, rather than any part within, is what critically matters in the art of transformation. Furthermore, when out-of-the-box possibilities are only mentioned in a smaller room, they gain little traction and easily dissipate. For something new to be introduced, experienced, and further sustained, a larger context must be built to host it. Only after the stage is made wider will more room for creative change become available.

The ecstatic healing traditions readily draw upon the performing arts to help awaken heightened emotion and its physical commotion. Perhaps better than anything else, music, song, and dance help expand the performance space required for healing. Conversation is minimized or may be entirely excluded. The custodians of the world's oldest living healing tradition, the Kalahari Bushmen of southern Africa, have healing sessions that involve no talk. Their healing ceremony starts with singing, clapping, and dancing. Only after this warm-up and its felt expansion of the ceremonial ground does healing commence. The client or patient is not limited to those requesting help—it is the whole community. Emotional fervor is needed to ignite the healer's body trembling and heightened singing that contribute to the healing means of tactile intervention. The Bushman word for this mix of strong emotion, somatic vibration, and its expression through song is *n/om*. Without the presence of *n/om* in a highly excited atmosphere and emotionally charged inner sphere, healing is not believed to be possible.

This kind of heightened emotion and intense ecstatic expression is obviously found missing in both psychotherapy and most contemporary healing practices. While we do not naïvely recommend that therapists build a fire and dance around it all night with clients, we are going to suggest that therapists acknowledge a broader performance stage that is open to the practical wisdom of elder healing traditions. Here therapists can learn how to tap into more excitement and increased emotion as a valuable resource. Whereas the Bushmen heal with extreme emotion and physical commotion, psychotherapy is usually extremely unemotional, with a guarded expression that keeps everyone in their chairs and a conversational tone that is seldom altered. From the onset, toned-down emotion and constrained expression are encouraged and even exalted. This calm and relaxed state holds back the room's expansion, leaving a session feeling emotionally cold and more creatively dead than alive. To bring forth the aliveness that makes creative therapy less humdrum than schooled and theoretically ruled therapy requires some degree of changed emotion, fervor, and inner fire on the part of the therapist. It takes a creatively plugged-in practitioner to awaken a potent session.

Once an ecstatically charged healing session has been experienced, most clinical work feels frightfully dead and boring. No matter how educated or trained the practitioner, it is the absence of a wide range of expression, the paucity of elevated emotion, and the lack of creative vitality that marks therapy as missing what is prevalent in traditional healing. After dancing with the Bushmen, shaking with the Caribbean shakers, and singing with Amazonian shamans, it makes less sense to calmly chatter with recycled patter in a session where people are in great need of awakening everything within and without that may help activate change.

Some ecstatic healing traditions excite the room and its participants better than others, that is, they have more practical know-how in how to activate the process of transformation. Our fieldwork identified the ecstatic lineages with this practical wisdom and we studied how each brings something unique to the mix. This led to our creation of what we call "Sacred Ecstatics," a syncretic blend of the pragmatics behind ecstatic healing and transformative change that is called "spiritual cooking" by many of its proponents. This metaphor speaks to the literal and metaphorical increase of emotional warmth that is experienced when the room expands for a session to creatively wake up.

In addition to Brad's former involvement with and study of diverse healing traditions, he worked with renowned body workers throughout the world and found that master body workers were as rare and difficult to find as master therapists and master healers. He concluded that all master practitioners, no matter their classified name, share this way of working: they always lean more toward improvisation than the replication of a standardized procedure. Brad introduced early versions of our creative approach to some of these leaders of contemporary healing and received enthusiastic endorsements. For instance, Dr. John Upledger, a founder of craniosacral therapy, wrote: "This work takes you straight to the core." Renowned physician, Dr. Robert Fulford, added his evaluation: "I personally experienced Keeney's work and believe it is the most direct path to healing and spiritual growth."

During this time Brad and Betty Alice Erickson (2006) wrote a biographical book entitled, *Milton H. Erickson: An American Healer.* Erickson's improvisational approach, guided by ongoing interaction with the client, was unlike the template approach of other therapists with the exception of Whitaker and his non-theoretical, experiential orientation. In the world of therapy two giants stood above the others—Milton Erickson and Carl Whitaker. Erickson was the master of improvising action for change and Whitaker widened the range of expression in therapeutic performance. Together they would have been quite the co-therapy team. Creative therapy, in a certain sense, incorporates the different sides that each of these therapists brought to the profession—improvisation and wider performance expression that aims to awaken a session and promote change.

Creative therapy's development also benefited from the contribution of a few other therapists. Salvador Minuchin (who regarded Whitaker as the only genius of psychotherapy) had amazing performance chops and was only limited by the structural family therapy model he always imposed—it could inspire or inhibit creative action. Few people could convey the confidence and healing assurance that Minuchin did in his sessions, a quality that was later criticized by more timid therapists who lacked his stage presence, systemic wisdom, and interactional skill. Minuchin invited Brad to teach at the Philadelphia Child Guidance Clinic where he was joined by Carl Whitaker for a brief time. Olga Silverstein was also an incredible agent of change and when she was tuned in, transformation would follow. She was affectionately regarded as a "witch" by some therapists who watched her live sessions. Brad, serving as Director of Research at the Ackerman Institute for Family Therapy where Olga worked as a clinician, wrote a book with her that analyzed a whole case she conducted (Keeney with Silverstein, 1986).

Like Whitaker, Olga regarded herself as non-theoretical and more intuitive, and like Erickson she preferred indirect intervention to trigger change. Brad's research at Ackerman focused on observing the therapeutic work of leading clinicians throughout the world with a preliminary, but not yet fully formed version of RFA. He had rare open access to therapists who saw him as a model-free, unbiased theoretician and an astute communication analyst. Competing therapists who sometimes wouldn't speak to one another had no issue inviting Brad to watch them work and talk about it afterwards.

Before retiring from fieldwork with renowned therapists, contemporary complementary medicine practitioners, and traditional healers, Brad had been authorized by Japanese healer Ikuko Osumi Sensei to oversee the future of authorized training associated with *seiki jutsu*, which translates as "the art of the vital life force." She regarded him as inheriting the legacy of her healing way. In the Kalahari, the elder Bushmen Brad had danced with for several decades recognized him as having equal power as a *n/om-kxao* (their name for healer or doctor), something confirmed by the former Harvard anthropologist and long-term anthropologist of Bushman culture, Megan Biesele. In St. Vincent and the Grenadines, Brad was anointed as a "spiritual captain." He was similarly welcomed in his local sanctified black church. Other traditions also adopted him into their spiritual and medicine ways including the Lakota, Ojibway, and Diné. He was fully initiated as a Balian healer in Bali, a grandfather shaman among the Guarani Indians, a sangoma and high sanusi among the Zulu, and recognized and accepted as a traditional spiritual healer in Mexico, Brazil, and Paraguay, among other places and traditions. After all these immersions into global spiritual ways and contemporary healing, bodywork, and therapy, we regard all of this transformative work as housed within the context of what we call "Sacred Ecstatics." The creative therapist in practice is someone who also benefits from the study and practice of healing traditions that have existed for thousands of years, with more enduring ancient wisdom than the relative infancy of psychotherapy and its "talking cure." Here you find that even a slight increase in the range of emotion and expression can dramatically boost a therapist's resourcefulness and provide an immediate escape from any model that holds back such change.

Early in his career, Brad found it difficult to share what he had learned about cybernetics, performance art, and healing to other therapists. He experienced most professional organizations, leaders, and teachers as having fallen into a frozen state, what we call the global cooling of the helping professions. They lack awareness and knowledge about how to warm a session and bring it to creative life. He found a reignited appreciation for Whitaker who he remembered would also sometimes sing in sessions as well as engage in all kinds of absurd performance. Brad found the same frustration that Whitaker lamented when trying to explain the importance of igniting a session with creative vitality. Brad considered quitting the psychotherapy profession numerous times and, on several occasions, purchased one-way airline tickets to faraway places, imagining he would not return.

Hillary and Brad Join Forces

All this changed when Hillary came into Brad's life. We were assigned to teach a graduate class together and Hillary's creativity, curiosity, appreciation for absurdity, and intellect immediately inspired him. She readily and clearly grasped the complexity and subtle nuance of cybernetics and recognized what was fundamental about his way of doing therapy. Together we invented a new kind of creative pedagogy in which the course invented itself as it went along and didn't know its subject matter until the end, after it was created. In other words, our course resembled a creative therapy session. This kind of teaching, called "circular poetics" by Hillary, was like creative therapy—an improvised performance art. Brad's motivation to teach was immediately rekindled.

Hillary recognized the importance of Brad's unfinished work with creative therapy and its contribution to clarifying and extending the transformative arts. With careful detective work she uncovered how cybernetic ideas had been historically misconstrued and misunderstood by the profession of family therapy and even cybernetics, especially when it forgot that cybernetics must include the "cybernetics of cyberneticians."[1] Her first book, *Circular Therapeutics: Giving Therapy a Healing Heart* (Keeney, 2012a), was an antidote to the proliferation of therapy models that exalted interpretation with a blind spot to interactivity and performance. *Circular Therapeutics* was critically praised by the major contemporary scholar of cybernetics, Klaus Krippendorff, Gregory Bateson Professor of Cybernetics, Language, and Culture at the University of Pennsylvania, as "an amazing work that exceeds the promise of Gregory Bateson's writing." *Circular Therapeutics* provided freshly tilled ground for the further growth of creative therapy, enabling it to make even more meaningful contact with the ancient healing arts.

Under Hillary's creative leadership, we built an experimental doctoral program in "creative systemic studies" (a name we invented) that tried to surpass disciplinary and interdisciplinary boundaries, offering more open means and ways of scholarly inquiry and transformational practice. We situated it in a state university's family therapy program and though we had relative independence from its administration, we discovered how context or the "room" in which one situates the work is more critical than we had ever imagined. Hillary continued to study how the helping professions, including family therapy, could so easily become iatrogenic or pathology inducing in spite of good intentions. They were simply too organized by perpetuating concretized institutionalized forms that impede the needed further development of change-oriented practice, pedagogy, and exploration of the art of transformation. We found ourselves constantly pushing back these forces of trivialization, whether it came from a student focused on passing a licensing exam, a professor maintaining the status quo, or an academic administrator only interested in exercising power over others.

Similarly, when we made keynote presentations at psychotherapy conferences or gave workshops to therapists, we encountered too many people more invested in preserving their allegiance to schools of therapy rather than advancing the art of change that includes changing themselves. Sometimes we felt we were talking to cult members who parroted clichés with no idea what they were actually saying or doing, or why. Each school of therapy seemed to follow the same trajectory noted in the history of religions—they start with creative inspiration and then quickly deteriorate into being a bureaucracy where people compete for a social role rather than foster its creative advancement.

In spite of this state of affairs, we decided to detail how a therapist could actually learn to become a creative facilitator of change rather than remain stuck in a theoretical model whose action primarily served self-verifying the model instead of helping anyone. Together we completed specifying the cybernetic groundwork that inspired creative therapy. We also finished laying out the pioneering method of RFA that shows how to construct a big room for transformation.

The performance of creative therapy along with specification of some of its operations was further advanced in our books, *Circular Therapeutics: Giving Therapy a Healing Heart* (2012a), *Creative Therapeutic Technique: Skills for the Art of Bringing Forth Change* (2013), and *Recursive Frame Analysis: A Qualitative Research Method for Mapping Change-Oriented Discourse* (2015). This work was accomplished during a time when we founded and directed the doctoral program in Creative Systemic Studies at the University of Louisiana. We also conducted work at several institutes that helped advance our work, particularly at the Central European Institute for Systemic Therapy in Budapest, Etfasis in Querétaro, Mexico and the University of Mexico in Mexico City. The books we published together, along with Brad's previous contributions, collectively provide practitioners with a radically different world-view or *weltanschauung* for the art of helping people change that spans practice, theory, training, and research. This body of work provides the background for the present volume that gives greater detail and prescriptive advice for the performance of a creative therapy session, a continuation of the previous book entitled, *The Creative Therapist: The Art of Awakening a Session* (Keeney, 2009).

Later in the midst of our early scholarly work together, Hillary met the Bushman elders who recognized her as a *n/om-kxao* and celebrated her natural talent for healing. She also formed a relationship with the daughter of the late Mother Ralph of St. Vincent, one of Brad's close spiritual colleagues.

She encouraged Hillary to further advance on the spiritual healing path. After being thoroughly "cooked" as a teacher and practitioner of ecstatic healing in its diverse forms, Hillary administered seiki and n/om (the Ju'/hoan Bushman word for seiki) to those studying its transformative way. Like Brad, Hillary recognized the importance of building a room for creative therapy practice that is big enough to hold creativity, performance art, healing, and the ineffable.

As a dancer, Hillary was uniquely prepared to study ecstatic movement as a special art form organized by the shifting intensity of emotion. As Associate Editor of the academic journal, *Dance, Movement, and Spiritualities,* she examined how dynamics of circularity, improvisation, and healing intertwine in sacred dance contexts. Her research focused on what healing dancers were doing in ecstatic lineages, especially the Kalahari Bushmen. She recognized how spontaneous movement is made primary in the interaction between these healers and those they hope to heal.

In addition, Hillary's prior residence in a Zen monastery prepared her to be resistant to exaggeration and tangential diversion in her descriptive accounts and in her action, preferring to point to what is most essential with the least distraction. The combination of her expertise with body movement and familiarity with an ancient practice that exercised clarity over obfuscation helped her discern what was important in the enactment of change in healing sessions. Hillary's gifts made her multi-tooled and well prepared to become the co-inventor of creative therapy and its contextualization in Sacred Ecstatics. Following Carl Whitaker's insistence on co-therapy over solo therapy, we formed a dedicated partnership whose combined resources created a more expansive therapeutic presence than either of us could accomplish alone.

Emergence of Sacred Ecstatics, the Context of Creative Therapy

We made the decision to leave academia in 2014 and establish new territory for the transformative arts. Rather than only add another therapeutic model to the present context that hosts practice, we decided that a radically expanded context was more needed. Going past the present contextual forms that house therapy, counseling, coaching, bodywork, and even contemporary healing meant building a different kind of space for helping people. We emphasized what is usually overlooked—that building a big room is more important than doing things differently inside the same constrained spaces maintained by the established therapy schools. We stopped teaching, presenting, and conducting sessions in small room contexts.

Our goal then was to more explicitly construct a performance space expansive enough to activate more emotion and creative expression in a session, including what takes place in the most powerful transformative practices we had personally encountered among ecstatic healers. It's important to interject that Brad had already for many years conducted sessions in clinics and at conferences all over the world as a kind of double agent. He performed as a therapist while secretly standing inside a different existential space, one that belonged both to the world of healing mystery and to the creative performing arts. He found that this enabled him to become more resourceful, creative, and therapeutic. As any traditional healer will tell you, it's nearly impossible to inspire change in someone else unless you yourself are plugged into your primary sources of inspiration. Despite Brad's ability to do masterful sessions, even in the most creatively dead spaces, at some point we both grew impatient with the unnecessary constraints that usually contextualize psychotherapy. Emboldened by our partnership, as well as encouraged by the colleagues and students who were moved by our sessions, we became more explicit about what kind of context better organizes and inspires this work.

We began to describe creative therapy as a process of ongoing existential expansion where the words spoken, and all the other action taken matter less than the context within which they are performed. We echoed what earlier systemic therapists had called for, but we were equipped with more tools to help specify and enact it. RFA enabled us to better discern how a larger context is built up over the course of a session rather than assumed to exist by merely mentioning certain metaphors once or twice. For instance, a therapeutic "reframe" isn't a reframe when first introduced; it is only a single utterance that has to be repeatedly re-indicated and extended until it is built up enough to become a frame that can hold other content. Otherwise, the initial "reframe" is only new content inside the same old frame. A big room unique to each session is built one metaphor at a time, weaving them together so the connections expand rather than reduce, becoming a web that hosts more variation and change. Rather than arrive with a conceptual filter that screens everything except the cherished ideas and spoken lines of a therapy model—whether it is a problem, solution, cognition, behavioral sequence, narrative, interpretation, or whatever—we arrive on an empty stage that we work to further expand until a surprise is brought to everyone, including us.

We decided to call the room of our work "Sacred Ecstatics" because it enabled us to hold the metaphors, names, and forms we find inspiring and useful, including "creative therapy," "circular therapeutics," "ecstatic healing," "improvisation," "performance," "theater of transformation," and the like. We now had the name of the big room along with the construction tool kit of recursive frame analysis but had not yet figured out how to teach the other necessary operations behind the art of creative therapy. Established therapy metaphors and concepts were too laden with the limitations we were trying to help others escape.

We headed to Budapest, Hungary where Dr. Dezsoe Birkas invited us to teach a two-week long master class in healing. We saw two cases each morning and two in the afternoon. The clients brought a wide range of presenting issues and more than a few had been diagnosed with schizophrenia. These sessions were observed by a group of therapists and other professional people helpers, including the psychiatric director of mental health services for Hungary. This event proved to be a turning point in our professional lives. The challenge was not in conducting the sessions but in teaching and describing our work to others without using terms that dragged in the antithetical baggage of psychotherapy. Again, using the latter's terms carried the liability that students would think we were making reference to conceptual understandings we actually wanted to avoid. We previously had to constantly qualify and often negate the metaphors we used to describe our work, and this made us as frustrated as our perplexed students. We realized that we had to create our own terms and glossary in order to more clearly specify our framework. We had to better speak about how to build a room big enough to hold, sustain, and further grow the practice of creative therapy.

Assuming that further intellectual precision would better specify our work, we were surprised that guidance would come from dreams. While Brad was no stranger to having visionary dreams, which had been a part of his previous fieldwork with traditional healers, we never expected to experience dreams that provided the descriptive metaphors that would make creative therapy more explicit. However, we aren't the first to create a therapy whose formation was influenced by dreams. The same happened to Carl Jung whose autobiographical account of encountering his unconscious demonstrates how dreams can powerfully shape therapy's language and design. When we thought about dreams from a creative therapy perspective, we realized that the expanded space of our sought "big room" belongs to what is not yet conscious and is therefore only accessible to the unconscious mind. This also explains the difficulty in trying to indicate what is unknown to others when the terms used are too familiar. Our sincere and passionate quest to reach into less familiar therapeutic territory must have naturally triggered the unconscious communication of dream.

From the first day of the Budapest master class, we started dreaming up various ideas and strategies that became the building blocks for a broader way of contextualizing creative therapy. The first cornerstone that was dreamed was the image of a "thermometer," a metaphorical way of indicating the "temperature" of a session. Ecstatic healing traditions, especially those in the African diaspora, speak of "hot" and "cold" when it comes to what they believe is the most important experiential quality in their ceremonies. When things are hot they are ecstatic—heightened emotion and somatic excitation are in operation, and if hot enough, the participants get "cooked," their name for the sought outcome of transformation. After this dream, we immediately recognized what was most absent in the sessions of the helping professions was what ecstatic healers call "heat"—both the feeling and expression of intense emotion that evokes awe, wonder, and excitement. Ecstatic experience is what breaks through the shrunken conceptual encapsulation of an impoverished life and enables a reset of the whole mind and body, especially concerning its spectrum of experience and expression. The concept of a thermometer registering the temperature of a session was the first contribution to building a vocabulary that better articulates the different kind of operations, dynamics, and changes that take place in creative therapy sessions.

When we returned from Budapest, we started a mentorship program and introduced our unique kind of creative session with its emerging vocabulary. We wrote the book, *Sacred Ecstatics: The Recipe for Setting Your Soul on Fire* (The Keeneys, 2016) and several other volumes that carefully describe and prescribe the context that we call a "big room" for our practice to reside within. In addition to presenting the construction know-how for building a room, we highlighted the other operations that help make a session "cook" and send a client home better equipped for change. We were finally able to provide a definition of creative therapy as a performing transformative art that benefits from (1) drawing upon the pragmatics of cybernetics that inspires change-focused action through a circular process rather than naively enacted lineal causality; (2) utilizing a wider of range of expression provided by the performing arts; and (3) learning practical wisdom from the older healing traditions that have expertise in the awakening and amplification of emotion that helps activate a more engaging experience of change.

The Re-Birth of the Creative Therapist

A common metaphor for cybernetics is Ouroboros, the mythical snake that swallows its own tail, re-creating itself through ongoing recursion. Each time it completes a round it emerges changed. The historical development of creative therapy has itself been an Ouroborean journey—the "therapy of therapy" Brad called for early in his career. Continuously submitting creative therapy to its own operations meant that its form and metaphors had to be open to change and so did we. Such roundabout improvisation constantly brings new resources to our work, all brought to life through experimental therapeutic action. This is the dynamic path of the creative therapist and the expanding stage for its circular therapeutics.

We now recognize that there is no limit to how vast the room of creative therapy can be and that the roles of therapist, performer, and healer easily overlap and morph. Any former separations between creative therapy, aesthetic performance, and ecstatic healing have been mended and wholly re-blended. As scholars, we remain rooted in the basic ideas of recursive process (the circularity of circularity) and especially its embodiment that was postulated by cybernetics. We still embrace the performing arts whose wide range of expression brings more means of evoking change. What lifts creative therapy to the next level is the more explicit incorporation of traditional healing whose elevated emotion leads to the indefinable, but experience-able creative force. When a creative therapy session dances with traditional healing ways, it does not lose its circular guidance or its respect for cultivating performance skill. Instead, it lands in a new frontier where the pragmatics of higher cybernetics, aesthetics, and ecstatics all contribute to altering the session room and everyone within it.

Please keep in mind that the sessions in this book still walk through the three-act theatrical play as creative therapy did before. They continue to emphasize improvisation that resourcefully weaves together creative metaphors and themes to construct a new reality unique to every client and session—the main operation of act one. Here we will disclose more of what occurs when a session transitions from act one to act two. The main operation of the middle act is called "getting experientially cooked by change." This is when creative energy is felt percolating in the atmosphere. The session undergoes what we call a "creative melt," where metaphor overtakes literal meaning, concretized belief, and entrenched interpretation. If the temperature rises high enough, the therapist's voice becomes more musical and rhythmic in tone, as therapy crosses over into becoming a more obvious theatrical performance. If a session cooks even further, the operations more recognizable in traditional healing spontaneously arise, including ideomotor movement that leads to a physical vibration that is transferable to the client. Finally, the last act brings the main operation of a special prescription to the stage. The therapist assigns creative action that helps the client take their transformational experience into the everyday. The degree of room expansion, the intensity of cooked expression, and the form of the final intervention are never predetermined—like all improvised work it is something that arises out of the interactions of the participants.

Creative therapy continues to invite those involved with the helping professions to leave its small rooms and unchanging methodological forms behind. It stands behind the previously articulated "in-and-out-of-the-box musings" (Keeney, 2009) that sidestep contrived theoretical coherency and overly fixed method in favor of a growing list of inspirational (and sometimes contradictory) ideas that more effectively move a therapist to act rather than revere theoretical consistence and persistence. If you want to know what to do in creative therapy, then improvisationally act and afterwards notice the interactional reverberations. Do not be organized by proving you or your model of therapy offer the smartest, sharpest explanation on the planet. Be less concerned with recycling understanding and more involved with creating a breakthrough live performance. Use all of your gifts and this includes the rational as well as the irrational creative impulse. As Whitaker encouraged, the therapist must bring their own "craziness" to a session, the kind of craziness that is creatively productive rather than boringly reductive. Hunt for what inspires and ignore what tires.

Once the room is existentially big, more that is resourceful will come into play. We invite practitioners to reach for the creative performance that is not mentioned in the licensing exams. Creative therapy in practice cares the least about what a therapist or client philosophically or diagnostically believes is going on with a person's life. You come to a session ready to act and take a leap into the unknown where changing mystery rather than re-told history resides. Creative therapy provides a setting for clients and therapists to become reset, retuned, and reintroduced to a wider spectrum of experiential possibilities.

Note

1 This is a joke we make about the so-called "cybernetics of cybernetics" that tried to turn around cybernetics to include its own operations. However, it too often did not include the whole cybernetician, only the cybernetician's observing, which paradoxically kept them outside (observing) rather than fully (participating) inside the cybernetic loop.

2

WHAT'S DIFFERENT ABOUT THE CREATIVE THERAPIST?

Begin at the End

Creative therapy emphasizes a radically practical approach that is uncommonly atheoretical. Each session begins with intervening action rather than diagnostic knowing. Subsequent assessment is then limited to discerning the immediate effects of the last attempted elicitation of change. In other words, the creative therapist primarily acts to evoke an *experience* of change within the session and does not consciously rely on any abstract diagnostic, theoretical, or ideological understanding to guide intervention. This orientation, inspired by cybernetician and radical constructivist Heinz von Foerster, challenges the common sense that holds back change-oriented action until more is clinically known about the client. We are taught to believe that we must first understand before we dare step into the action stream. This is the well-worn clinical path that moves from clinical assessment to treatment strategy. Creative therapy flips this temporal arrangement, placing action ahead of knowing. It immediately aims to change the present situation and then follows up with another attempt at change, this time benefitting from the experienced outcome of the previous attempt.

It may be shocking to imagine abandoning the need to understand the client and that the knowing that matters during a session is improved know-how for the subsequent action that steadfastly aims for change, a noticed difference that is more sensed than measured. Here everyone in the room notices that the room feels different, that something happened or is starting to happen that was not present before. The creative therapist's diagnostic knowing is limited to discovering whether such change was experienced the moment the therapist acts to set it in motion. Creative therapy never asks the kind of questions or reviews psychological test results that lead to a psychiatric diagnostic label and then, on the basis of the gathered information, proceeds to select a pre-approved match of treatment plan. While this latter medical structure continues to heavily influence therapy, another genre of therapeutic practice was introduced decades ago. This alternative strategy distinguished creative improvisation from any therapy model that moves from theoretical cognition to therapeutic action (Keeney, 1991). Now called creative therapy, this improvisational orientation directly seeks experiential change through introducing and building upon the unexpected surprises, experienced transitions, and felt shifts that take place during a session.

The antiquated diagnostic nomenclature of psychiatry has been long contested as a fiction lacking any significant relevance other than serving the habit of labeling pathology, disabling creativity, and imposing social control. Thomas Szasz saw it as a category mistake that confused "problems in living" with "medical disease." In a 1958 issue of *Columbia Law Review* he argued that mental illness was a myth, an interpretation that was the equivalent to claiming possession by the devil (as cited in Oliver, 2006). Whitaker called diagnostic assessment "pornographic" because it forced clients to behave as exhibitionists while a therapist acted as a "peeping Tom." However, what is seldom critiqued is how diagnosis can shapeshift—when one diagnostic system is eliminated it is instantly replaced by another kind. For example, problem-focused therapists evaluate how a problem definition is related to descriptions of attempted solutions before designing an intervention. Similarly, solution-focused therapists assess the client's history of solutions and diagnostically scan the client's imagination for possible alternatives in a fantasized miraculous future. Family therapists may diagnose the family structure, present state of relationships, historical constellations, conversational content, and dyadic, triadic, schismatic, or homeostatic dynamics before trying to change a malfunction. When it comes to diagnosis, "birds do it, bees do it, even educated fleas do it," and even narrative therapists do it, that is, they critically inspect a client's narrative to spot its errors or contaminants before acting with the client to edit it. Last but not diagnostically least, postmodern therapists with an allergy to any strategy of change continuously diagnosis the therapist to make sure there is no appearance of purposeful intervention, preferring another style of conversation as an implicit means of change. When thoroughly examined, all therapies seem unable to avoid starting without some kind of hypothetical knowing that involves assessment, diagnosis, and theoretical interpretation, whether of the brain, the psyche, problems, solutions, behavioral habits, cognitive maps, narratives, family systems, cultural beliefs, postmodern sentiments, conversational styles, and all the other thematic subjects of interest. While creative therapy always assesses, it takes place *after* rather than before each therapeutic effort to stir up an experience of change, and only evaluates what can help improve the next effort. This is what makes it so unique and different from the get-go.

What does a session look like that begins with raw action rather than hunts for elaborated understanding? In one session our first spoken line invited the client to leave the office and take a ten-minute walk outside. The client was instructed to make the change they desired during this odyssey and to not wait any longer. We advised that the walk to change should be done as if the client's entire future depended on it. Before the departure, we mentioned that the outside environment might have some surprising material objects on the ground that offer a hint at what could help resolve, dissolve, or evolve their situation. A tree branch, acorn, piece of paper, stone, feather, old toy, blade of grass, pencil, leaf, lost part, loose change, or anything at all might be found that, with a little bit of help from the client's intuition and imagination, could be regarded as a possible sign for how to move forward. The client was then instructed to bring whatever treasure was found back to the office. Without any further conversation, we stood up, opened the door, and announced, "We'll see you in ten minutes and we look forward to welcoming and celebrating your change."

This is one example of how a creative therapy session can begin. It starts with an intervention that offers a difference and then determines if it made a difference—a therapeutic act that primes the pump of change. It then works with the outcome that ensues. If the client comes back with a rock, then this is accepted as a primary metaphor that helps guide the session. Other related metaphors and themes can follow like "unbreakable," "strength," "solidity," "well-worn," "smooth," "dense," "erosion," "ancient," "diamond-in-the-rough," "hidden designs not obvious until closely observed," and so forth. As this conversation advances, it never leaves the rock behind. It remains a foundational metaphor on which the room or context of the session is built. Perhaps it leads to exploring a theme neither therapist nor client ever anticipated. The exemplary session here might finally address the mineralogy of life, the boulders that hold one up, the way flat rocks are better designed to skip on water while well-rounded rocks do a better job of sinking to the bottom, or how "Rocky" was a movie that showed how hope and hard work can bring about a seemingly impossible victory. It can even lead to discovering other creative therapists who use rocks in their sessions as Brad and his home visit team did in the Delta region of Louisiana (Keeney, Lawson, & Roose, 2010).

In a very real sense, creative therapy begins where other therapies think they should end. Its first move is an intervention that can include an elaborated drama about selecting which chair to sit in: "Before you sit down, we'd like to know whether you prefer sitting on a soft or hard surface, or whether the color and design of the chair could influence what you say today. We once had a client who sat on a blue pillow and she couldn't stop talking about pie in the sky." Everything said by the therapist and the client is connoted as an intervention—a wild shot in the dark that leads to other trial-and-error shots that gradually lead you nearer to hitting the target. The aimed for bullseye is never anything less than a *bona fide* experience of change. We are referring to the kind of changed outcome that fascinates, excites, and expands the client's phenomenal world. The very elicitation of any unexpected experience in the session is itself the embodiment of such change.

Treat the Room, Not the Client

As the session moves along the change highway, the creative therapist aims for ever-increasing contextual expansion. Improvisation does not foster a mindless and goalless "anything goes" performance. It is undoubtedly outcome oriented, using what arises in the interaction to advance the session along a trajectory that expands the context so it can hold a vaster spectrum of experience. As we will soon elaborate, the "existential room" itself and its "climate" are what a creative therapist treats and tries to change. The agent of change is the changing interaction of therapist and client, not the solo therapist (or any "treatment factor") in vitro. The therapist and client surprise, trip, and reinvent one another rather than reenact a mundane performance of recycled therapeutic clichés, formerly rehearsed scripts, and predetermined roles. This provides the means for making the room big enough and the climate favorable enough for learning, growth, and transformation to take place.

Since creative therapy regards itself as a performing art rather than an applied social science or medical treatment, it is the world of performance to which we turn for its structure. As described before (Keeney, 2009), each creative therapy session is regarded as a three-act play with a beginning act, a middle act, and a final ending act. The first sought outcome of a creative therapy session takes place in act one and it is bold: here we wish to change the entire reality of a client. We call this operation "building a big room." Rather than only attempt to alter an attitude, thought, myth, action, pattern of interaction, or relational system, the creative therapist hopes to change the whole kit and caboodle. In other words, the room, the stage, and the theater of the client's performed life are blown wide open with the former walls and ceiling removed so any part, dimension, or quality is freer to move about with more space for the appearance of other previously unnoticed resources. For example, the client in the previous example might find that rocks are more interesting to look at than reading self-help psychology books or watching Dr. Phil, the television therapist. Or a rock collection might get underway with a stone gathered each time the client is able to hold a boundary and not cave in to others.

Creative therapists have a trade secret missed or forgotten by others. They know that when a change occurs within the same contextual room in which the client is accustomed to living, it does not provide much of a difference. The sought change moves the client outside the previous walls that confined and defined the range of possible experience. Therapists who insist on seeing whole family systems rather than any of its isolated individual members may already have a taste of this expansion—as long as they help broaden rather than shrink the family room. When Brad directed clinical doctoral programs he sometimes designated different treatment rooms to host the progressive changes a family experienced in a session. By the end of the therapeutic hour, they would have sat in at least three rooms, marking the beginning, middle, and end of the therapeutic journey. He also experimented with changing the degree of lighting to mark these room transitions—a session started in the dark and got brighter as the therapeutic context expanded. Of course, the existential room does not need to be associated with changes in a physical space or its theatrical illumination. Any room will automatically feel different, changed, and more inclusive of a larger territory when a shift from one act to another is made. Everyone will experience it, even observers behind a one-way mirror.

Creative Therapy Is Outcome-Based Throughout the Session

We regard creative therapy as the most outcome-oriented therapy possible. This is because the therapist is perceptually attuned to the outcome of each action in a session—the experiential impact it has on others, including the therapist. This outcome, as we discuss it in the next chapter, is something that must be perceived by the senses—seen, heard, smelled, tasted, or felt—rather than theoretically hypothesized or statistically calculated. The experienced micro-outcomes that take place throughout a session are what steadily steer a session forward, rather than any post hoc analysis of a single session or series of sessions. The time to assess therapy is when it is happening rather than afterwards when the experienced moments are lost. The idea that a "whole session" or an "entire therapy" can be measured is itself a mistake in misplaced concreteness that confounds levels of logical description.[1] The further an evaluation is distanced from the actual lines uttered and the experiences evoked, the less trustworthy, meaningful, or useful it is for helping better guide a subsequent performance.

The creative therapist relies upon the many ongoing outcomes that occur during a session and finds that any construed assessment of the summation of a whole session by quantitative means is more an indication of social science schizophrenia than representative of anything that experientially took place. Watching a video or examining a whole unedited transcription afterwards provides more reliable empirical data than statistical numerology, in part because it reveals the whole sequence of interaction and how it unfolded over the course of a session (see Keeney, Keeney, & Chenail, 2015).

Finally, a creative therapy session is more like attending the theater where no one would be taken seriously if they used a psychological questionnaire or sociometric survey instrument to assess the outcome of the performance. At its best, a session is like a grand night at the theater that evokes an experience that touches and moves others in a profound manner. A session is either aesthetically dead or alive, which is a more reliable indication of existential significance.

The proof of the pudding is found in the taste experienced when eating, not in counting the number of bites taken or weighing the diner. If we ask a family whether they like grandmother's cake more than her cookies, pudding, or pie and notice them spring to life with curiosity and excitement, we have an outcome that we will immediately feed rather than ignore. If the family protests or is puzzled by the question in an interesting or emotionally charged way, this is also a useful outcome because the client's response brought some energetic life to the conversation. The outcome we value is one that alters the experiential climate as it expands what is possible to address in the session. However, any other studied outcome that ignores or cannot bring back an instant replay of the family's response to grandmother's desserts is unable to notice when, how, or whether a session experientially changed. It has no clue what specific contributing actions took place in what sequence or in what context. The creative therapist wisely ignores this kind of social science fiction data and its make-believe findings, recognizing that its primary goal and outcome are to expand the researcher's publication list but not the room that holds the performance of therapy.

The creative therapist arrives at each session ready to build a therapeutic reality that is capable of advancing change. The building materials (metaphors and their connective links) that will be used, and the emergent forms of the new reality are always a surprise and are only revealed as the session progresses from one act to the next. The effect of an attempted change of experience (not just a change of the "problem") is what steers the movement rather than a hypothetical generalization about the client's psycho-social-cultural state. The latter can only be gleaned by stepping out of an ongoing interaction, pausing to ponder and reflect—an interruption that risks interfering with and dulling what otherwise might be an exciting process of change that is in motion. The process-oriented assessment and continuous outcome-based action of creative therapy involve the same discernment found in other performing arts. The therapist relies on keen sensory awareness that especially includes an intuition or "feel" for when the room is creatively coming to life. This tacit know-how, formerly called clinical acumen, involves more feeling than thinking. Its gnosis "feels its way forward" while not knowing what is next in store. Sensory experience and intuition calibrate the self-correcting action of improvisation. Furthermore, such action and its follow-up evaluation happen almost instantaneously without the need to interrupt the flow. There is no reason to call a timeout to hypothesize what is happening in the room unless it naturally arises as a way of empowering the ongoing march toward change.

Pay More Attention to the Unexpected: The Cybernetic Walkabout

The creative therapist pays the least attention to the expected and instead is on the lookout for the unexpected in a session—that which lies outside the walls of a therapy model and the small room in which the client resides. More a treasure hunt than an archeological dig, creative therapy knows there is no map that provides a direct route to the treasure. Creative therapy moves around a self-correcting circle where each step guides the next step taken, based on sensing whether the room is getting bigger—something easier said than done.

This circular walkabout, formally known as cybernetics, was first introduced to the therapy profession by Gregory Bateson and further elucidated by Brad (Keeney, 1983), followed by more correction and elaboration by Hillary (H. Keeney & B. Keeney, 2012a). It provided a well-rounded alternative trajectory to those seeking relief from dead-end models that promise change based on knowing what you'll do before you start. Rather than reenact a priori expectations, the cybernetic walkabout chases the unexpected, the differences that elicit more differences—enacting the process of change. Cybernetics calls for a more creative therapist who improvises rather than memorizes therapeutic lines and protocols (Keeney, 1991; H. Keeney & B. Keeney, 2013).

In creative therapy, the therapeutic action taken to trigger change comes back full circle to itself become a target of change. Each outcome is used to guide the next step: this is the cybernetic walkabout. Rather than evaluate what is wrong with clients—whether it is their faulty genes, maladaptive learning, ineffective attempted solutions, impoverished narratives, or whatever—the creative therapist focuses on changing the therapist's action one step at a time. This "instant karma" approach recognizes and utilizes that whatever the therapist does will ricochet through the room and then boomerang back and hit the therapist in the head, thus calibrating the next interaction between therapist and client. This creative improvisational process emphasizes changing the therapist's action, class of action, and entire (class)room of interaction. Trial-and-error learning occurs through using rather than ignoring a perceived deviation or mistake, and this is the ongoing process of self-correction. Respect and incorporate the learning offered by an error so that the next step is better taken.

The creative therapist is always asking what can be done rather than what else needs to be known or understood about the client. It is better for the therapist to rein in the habit of listening to everything the client communicates so their sensory awareness is not so cluttered that they miss hearing, seeing, or feeling any important difference that arrives. "Difference" should be noticed above all, the kind of difference that inspires different action. Here is found creative therapy's change-oriented performance that acts in order to perpetuate a never-ending sequence of experienced differences, each evoking what is next forthcoming.

Creative therapy is rooted to the radical shift toward a cybernetic trajectory and guidance strategy that few therapists grasped during the heyday of early family therapy and brief therapy. The same lineal journey from diagnosis to intervention remained instead of jumping on the circular tracks. Rather than make the action-cognition flip and take the circular walkabout, therapists only substituted a formerly preferred interpretation with a newly preferred one. They then waited in each session until they were adequately informed before taking action that would bring the expected change. Even the "interactional view" and "systemic view" still emphasized taking a look before prescribing a change. The more that interpretation changed, the more a therapist remained a model-bound interpreter who too often missed making the adjustment that could have made a higher order difference.

It isn't easy learning how to get in front of the viewing rather than behind it. It's even more difficult to trust that a circular walkabout with the client is what moves a session forward. The pragmatic notion that went missing in action was this: the circular trajectory is also the session's wheel of therapeutic transportation. When it turns, everyone on board moves forward. Follow what is resourceful, unexpected, interesting, or outside the current cramped box and then keep following that direction so that change becomes the ongoing transport process rather than the sought ending.

Years ago, we had a colleague who was the former director of a renowned problem-focused brief therapy institute with a focus on the interactional view. Together we were members of a faculty committee assigned to evaluate a student's clinical work at a final exam. The student described a session with a woman who had passionately told her that during the previous week she had been showered with numerous, incredible experiences of owls. She had dreamed of an owl and then that same day one flew over her head. The client gave one incredible owl report after another, enough to inspire a short story writer or playwright. We asked the student how she utilized the owl in her session. Before she could answer, our colleague interrupted and announced that the owl was not important. He wanted to know what the problem definition was and what solutions had been attempted. His "interactional view" caused blindness to anything other than his preferred model and its focus on problems and solutions, so the owl as an extraordinary therapeutic metaphor was ignored. A creative therapist working more like Milton Erickson than his pals in Palo Alto would recognize that the owl was a gift to the session—an unexpected difference whose wings of creative inspiration could take them anywhere, including the outcome that enabled the therapist and supervisor to no longer give a hoot about any unchanging view. The creative therapist gets ahead of opaque theoretical filters that block recognizing what might inspire a one-of-a-kind session. As a final note, the meeting we described took place in our colleague's office where directly behind his chair on a bookshelf sat a porcelain figurine of an owl.

The generalized views and strategies offered by therapy models excommunicate the unexpected and thereby limit the scope of what can contribute to helping a session change. Therapists are taught to walk the lineal road from knowing to action rather than traverse the circular walkabout that improvises each unexpected step. When theoretical viewing guides therapeutic doing, there is less likelihood of any significant difference or surprise to arise as the practitioner only stares at a theoretical map that excludes unfamiliar and unexplored territory. This is an example of what cybernetician Heinz von Foerster called "the law of cognitive homeostasis." The therapist acts to maintain a preferred stable therapeutic reality via strict adherence to an unchanging model that prescribes an unchanging view. The latter is in turn further solidified by its corresponding unchanging habits of self-verifying action. In other words, there is no room and no permission to creatively work with rocks or owls if they are not on the map, even when they are stumbled upon or are sighted overhead in the territory.

Don't Trust the Anti-Action Propaganda

Once upon a time not so long ago, the name "cybernetics" was spotted by a handful of "systemic therapists," but much like the owl it was never allowed to make a difference that could have made a long-lasting pragmatic difference. The earliest rendition of cybernetics (also called "first-order cybernetics") heretically offered a liberating flight from theoretical plights caused by stabilized viewing that impedes altered doing. Almost as soon as one step toward cybernetics was attempted (explicitly by Paul Watzlawick, John Weakland, and Richard Fisch and implicitly by Jay Haley's communication orientation), the field stopped in its tracks and then slid back into the old cultural habit of placing interpretation before action. Cybernetics was appropriated as another interpretive lens rather than followed as a prescription for more circular therapeutic action. The paradigmatic leap *into* a circular therapeutic reality was never fully made, and thus there remains very little that is systemic or cybernetic in the performance of so-called "systemic therapy" (H. Keeney & B. Keeney, 2012c). Though we expect more than a few "systemic therapists" to disagree with our objection that they aren't as systemic as they and their heroes claim to be, Klaus Krippendorff, the Gregory Bateson Professor for Cybernetics, Language, and Culture at the University of Pennsylvania shares our evaluation of the profession: "When therapists discovered cybernetics, many started using its vocabulary without living up to its promises … [it missed] what cybernetics can do when actually embodied in practices of living, not merely talked about. It opposes following therapeutic theories and advocates instead surrendering one's preconceptions to an involvement in the kind of virtuous circularities that can bring forth learning, healing, and improvisation—not just for clients but, in the evenhanded spirit of cybernetics, for therapists as well." And finally, he advised "therapists [be] willing to overcome their entrapment in the theories of traditional schools … and [learn the] circular way of being in communication with one another."

The historical breakup of the former courtship of therapy with cybernetics is inseparable from what we have called the "Hoffman blunder" (H. Keeney & B. Keeney, 2012a). Lynn Hoffman (1993) presented an unfortunate distortion of both first-order and second-order cybernetics that was like a confusion technique or ideological grenade thrown into therapy discourse that sent it rolling back to the former days of interpretation. Hoffman celebrated second-order cybernetics as a paradigmatically new kind of "view" or "lens" that invited the therapist to be one step removed from the therapeutic interaction in order to self-reflect, interpret, and take less action to help change a client's situation. What Hoffman overlooked is that she took the same step backwards as the strategically oriented and systemically informed therapists she criticized. They all took a step back to observe. Some therapists first observed in order to invent tactical action for change while Hoffman and her like-minded colleagues observed in order to advance the action of interpreting, doing so with a prohibition against any other kind of tactical action. Hoffman's misunderstanding of second-order cybernetics as a theory that promotes removed observation and self-reflection was shared at the time by the Galveston team formerly headed by Harold Goolishian with Harlene Anderson by his side, and Hoffman credits them both for influencing her migration to interpretation.

Lynn Hoffman had been a close friend of Brad's when he worked at the Ackerman Institute in New York in the early 1980s. They regularly met for lunch and she would pick his brain about cybernetics, since Brad had emerged as the leading cybernetic theorist in family therapy with the publication of *Aesthetics of Change* (1983). He watched the whole drama unfold that began with her using cybernetics to establish her authority and then once it was secured, she redefined it to denounce its original definition, so she and her colleagues could bring back the primacy of interpretation while criticizing strategic action. This combination of rhetorical sophistry and scholarly mystification placed both cybernetics and clients on the couch again. Though Hoffman appeared meek as a sheep in person, her writing could have the teeth of a wolf eager to tear apart those the profession had formerly revered as masters of therapeutic change.

Hoffman's (1993) version of second-order cybernetics was a negation of all of cybernetics, a point we examine in more detail in *Circular Therapeutics*

(2012a). Others contributed to the unraveling of the cybernetic circle with their own versions of the Hoffman blunder, advancing the hegemonic narrative that misidentified cybernetics and Gregory Bateson as calling for the exaltation of interpretation and the exclusive handling of meaning (White & Epston, 1990). The complete turn away from circularly organized action toward another round of comparative interpretation was made as therapists stood in front of a mirror and asked, "Mirror, mirror on the wall, who has the fairest reflection and narrative of them all?" Harlene Anderson (1997) launched a vicious attack on first-order cybernetics and therapists associated with its ideas, claiming that they promoted patriarchy and encouraged therapists to treat human beings like machines. Anderson then also repeated Hoffman's erroneous claim that second-order cybernetics was a call to retreat from cybernetic action and therapeutic intervention. Painting a picture of strategically oriented therapists as misogynist, power-hungry puppeteers, Anderson's book was an anti-systemic, anti-cybernetic propaganda campaign cloaked in postmodern metaphors that were arguably more a modern translation than a reflection of postmodern sentiment and aesthetic. Perfumed with feel-good truisms about embracing multiple truths and welcoming diverse viewpoints, the relative popularity of postmodern therapy may also stem from the fact that systemic therapy models are more difficult to learn than an open-ended, meandering conversational approach.

A whole new generation of interpreters did the same—they interspersed their therapy orientations with unassailable platitudes and unclearly defined abstractions from scientific and philosophical traditions that few dared question lest they be seen as less educated or politically incorrect. As published therapists cut out and tossed around terms they did not understand, from Ilya Prigogine's "dissipative structures" to Humberto Maturana's "perturbations," therapists became more confused while being assured they had become more enlightened. Michael White's understanding of Foucault was summarized by the title of Luepnitz's (1992) paper, "Nothing in Common but Their First Names: The Case of Foucault and White." As she concluded, narrative therapy "attempts to authorize one clinician's work by dropping a few poorly understood terms from an erudite French philosopher. Nothing could be more anti-Foucauldian" (p. 284). In the midst of this social contagion of mystifying muddle, the field of family therapy suddenly was rife with missing bodies, absent families, lost interactions, and forbidden interventions, all replaced by the kind of talk that was inspired by propaganda patter and theoretical splatter.

Hoffman's and Anderson's idiosyncratic interpretations and alterations of both first- and second-order cybernetics would not even be worthy of mention had they not spread throughout the field like a confusion virus that persists to this day. It's unfortunate that more women with a better grasp of first- and second-order cybernetics did not loudly protest both postmodern and narrative therapists' conflation of cybernetics and systemic therapy with patriarchy and sexism (and racism and other forms of oppression). Whatever patriarchal values or sexist views may have been held by leading male systemic therapists at the time should not have been grounds for outright dismissal of either their contributions or the cybernetic theories that inspired them.

Rather than morally evaluate and readily reject a school of therapy based on hypothesized hidden agendas and presumed faulty ideologies, we advocate starting with a dramaturgical analysis of what is actually performed in a session using Recursive Frame Analysis (RFA). The creative therapist prefers using RFA to score a session instead of trying to settle any ideological or personal score with another therapist. The unfolding action in a session, including the words spoken, better reveal what takes place in therapy than an outside observer's filtered perception, theoretical translation, and biased interpretation of it. Before lauding or lambasting therapists' work let us first make clear what took place in a session, making sure we return to a replay of the performance to hear, see, and feel what the actors did and said and in what context. A performance is more representative of the therapy than what is later said about it via language and ideas that were never expressed in the session. The unacceptable cost of elevating interpretation over performance is that it enables the observer to claim that their interpretation rather than the event itself is more real. When only reflections are seen, the only view in the mirror is one that makes the observer supreme as the session is erased from memory.

The well-schooled creative therapist understands that second-order cybernetics encourages jumping *inside* the cybernetic circle to mutually influence and be co-influenced by a widened field of interaction. This surrender to being a part of the whole therapeutic ecology promotes a situational ethics that does not impose the therapists' ideological preferences for or against categories of action. To be one-step removed in order to better observe, reflect, and interpret while claiming "it's betta because it's meta" leaves the therapist ensnared in a peculiar entanglement. Again, the room set up by the extreme non-change agents like Hoffman and Anderson is the same space occupied by their fantasized and mythologized nemesis—the first-order cybernetics interventionist whose diagnose-then-act performance is also one-step removed from the observed system. Each theoretically opposed therapist occupies the same relationship to the client—one is worried that she will purposefully facilitate change and the other is concerned that she won't be as lucky.

Creative therapy brings back an old therapeutic wisdom adage: it asks *how*, not whether, therapists are participating to help or hinder change from taking place. Creative therapists do not filter the client's experience through an interpretive lens that is primarily meant to self-verify a model or ideology.

They cleanse the lens, clear the stage, get closer to the action, and start fresh with each session, more able and willing to creatively act in order to expand the room and change the way things change in order to enable more kinds of change.

Creative therapists apply the action-oriented, participatory wisdom of embodied second-order cybernetics that makes therapy models subject to their own operations of change. This "therapy of therapy" provides a "correction" of any stubborn idea, metaphor, behavioral habit, or technique. It can even result in editing the names of entrenched therapy models. Narrative therapy advances to plot therapy or dramaturgical therapy; problem-focused and solution-focused models converge into problem-solution or solution-problem interactional therapy; the interactional view becomes the interactional performance; postmodern therapy becomes more postmodern, reborn as labyrinths therapy, catch-22 therapy, or gravity's rainbow therapy, depending on the shifting (rather than perpetually bland) mood of the postmodernist; and finally cybernetic therapy becomes creative therapy that is free to roam in a room big enough to include all the others as they come and go in response to the unique circumstances at hand. Creative therapists move closer to the process of change rather than further away, where they become out of focus and out of touch with the experienced dynamics of transformation, lost in a house of reflective mirrors.

More Unconscious Involvement and Less Conscious Interference

Creative therapy has several beloved heroes of therapy who on the surface may appear to be opposites, but with a deeper examination are found to be complements who draw from the same source of wisdom. By now it is no surprise to hear that Carl Whitaker and Milton Erickson are two of creative therapy's guiding stars. Both were less driven by theory and preferred to evoke an experience of change. These therapists trusted the unconscious within themselves and others more than they did consciously driven communication, whether it involved talk or nonverbal action.

Whitaker and Erickson were not interpreters of the unconscious psyche like Freud or Jung whose approaches left the embodied and performed dynamics of the unconscious behind, replacing it with a verbal translation for conscious consideration. The conversion of unconscious ore into a theoretical gem is the interpretive therapists' talking cure fantasy. However, Erickson and Whitaker chose not to go spelunking in unconscious caves to retrieve lost problematic influences and then bring them into conscious light for release, comparable to exposing troublesome vampires to the sun. They regarded the unconscious as a treasure chest instead of a Pandora's box, filled with wisdom that can enrich and guide the process of change. Instead of elevating the translation of unconscious process into conscious content, they banned the conscious from distorting, diluting, or deleting unconscious wisdom through any narrative means of translation that renders a second edition one giant step removed from its primary source.

Erickson and Whitaker belonged to the greater community of healers who tacitly followed their own unconscious lead and refused to make it subservient to explicit interpretations, maps, and models. They had the least trust in derivative knowing and placed their therapeutic bet on the innate wisdom that surpasses what can be cognitively computed and interpreted. These unpredictable performers of the therapy stage were considered outsiders to the rest of the profession. Both of them relied on unconscious creativity. The unconscious, lest no one ever forget, hosts raw analogical and digitally illogical experience untouched by conscious narration's translated filtration. The unconscious is felt as something unexplainable that inspires unplanned action, which itself is the unexpected change that expands the therapy room.

The ongoing outcome-based orientation we previously described relies on less conscious discernment. Clinical acumen resides in the unconscious and is more somatically felt than thought. Whitaker and Erickson followed their gut and heart, with a disciplined mind obedient to both. Creative therapy values unconscious wisdom that has the practical street smarts to keep the conscious from interfering with its guidance of the interaction. Sessions are journeys into the unknown led by seeking what feels refreshingly unfamiliar because this is what unexpected change feels like. Here the computations of the unconscious follow the algorithms of the heart not the ratiocinations of mind.

The difference between the unconscious and conscious is an analog of the difference between an experienced performance and any post hoc construed knowing about it. Insight of any kind—psychoanalytic or interactional—does not only cause blindness as Paul Watzlawick humorously claimed. More importantly, it renders the therapist out of touch with the unconscious. Too much emphasis on theoretically filtered sight blocks the line of communication from the unconscious to the conscious and makes the latter supreme while disqualifying dream, intuition, and even a surprising, unexpected owl. What the offspring of Erickson missed, from the Mental Research Institute to Steve de Shazer's miracle cliché and NLP's cartography, was that subjecting Erickson's work to more conscious explanation and routinized technique disconnected it from the important operations of the unconscious that were at the heart of his work. Erickson discovered that the unconscious, the former alchemist's *pleroma* that entranced both Jung and Bateson, reigns under and over all that can be known and mapped. When this essential truth is missed, so is the essence of Erickson's art. In the unconscious is found the performance art and its aesthetics of change, as Brad suggested years ago (Keeney, 1983).

Whitaker radically proclaimed that without the therapist's unconscious "craziness" having its say, a session would be dead and a sheer waste of time.

He avoided and despised theories, techniques, and models for therapeutic conduct whose overly conscious knowing assured that a session would be boring (Whitaker, 1976). Whitaker told Brad that dependency on a therapy model drains the "blood" out of a therapist, leaving them existentially empty. While he considered the conscious mind to be absurd and found the unconscious to make more therapeutic sense, Erickson sought the unconscious trance that could help enhance the dance with change. It is important to not miss the fact that Erickson's therapeutic hypnosis was first applied to himself, making him less distracted by his own body pain (due to polio) as well as helping him be less influenced by the inner and outer conversational noise that would block his ability to hear and see between the lines. His hypnosis acted to expand the levels of communicational complexity, not restrict the focus to a singularity. Like Mozart, Erickson worked in the weave of counterpoint rather than over-emphasized consciously making a point. In his hypnotic mix, the unconscious could better fix whatever troubling muddle the conscious self had gotten itself into.

Neither Erickson nor Whitaker analyzed the dreams of their clients, but Whitaker sometimes fell asleep and dreamed during a session. When he woke up he shared it as an intervention to wake up the session. The un-interpreted dream could then continue to dream, that is, allow the unconscious to further express itself in the room. What's important here is that Whitaker's waking dream state and Erickson's altered trance state did not dissociate them from the client—they were brought a step closer into the system. The difference between their genius and that of others who tried to approximate it is that they were pulled more inside the ongoing interactions rather than thrown outside it for observation. Rather than wanting therapy to be more observer-able, they preferred making it more changeable. The first live session of therapy Brad ever watched was conducted by Whitaker who partially dozed off and then said to the father of the family, "I just dreamed you were a frozen block of ice." The family started laughing before the father could respond, "I'm in the refrigeration business." Awakened by this unconsciously produced metaphor, the rest of the session helped thaw the whole family.

Carl Whitaker brought a wider range of performance to his sessions than may have ever been seen before—he fell asleep, wrestled with clients, read the newspaper, spoke nonsense, and did his best to act crazier than his clients did, resulting in more room for the client to help normalize him. Erickson, who also enjoyed a healthy dose of nonsense talk, was more physically limited to using his voice because he was in a wheelchair. He became a master cryptologist and illogicologist who sent secret messages to the client's unconscious by an interspersed metaphor that made no sense on the surface but could be internally heard knocking on the unconscious door. He would appear to be talking to the conscious when he was actually only distracting it, utilizing one metaphorical phrase as a Trojan horse with another message for the unconscious hidden inside. Whether through crazy action, nonsense, absurdity, illogical logic, or coded multi-tiered talk, the unconscious was accessed and brought into the interactions with the client. Whatever ensued was then immediately utilized to weave an alternative reality where the unconscious could communicate while the conscious mind took a nap rather than imposed a map.

The creative therapist trusts the outcomes detected by a finely tuned unconscious, never relying on a consciously derived measure that madly pretends to be more objective because it eliminates sensory experience and intuition. When the therapeutic unconscious wakes up, the senses are actually further heightened and more able to notice what is happening in the moment. This may seem paradoxical: to better notice what's going on around you, invite the unconscious to participate. To do this the creative therapist must restrain the conscious mind and its cognitive homeostatic habits that ignore emotions, body sensations, and filter out unexpected or out-of-frame communication that might upset its apple cart. Again, this requires rejecting the common imperative to listen more "actively" to clients in order to better understand their situation. Consciously trying to discern some underlying coherence in a client's communication just imposes the therapist's way of construing meaning, getting everyone more lost in interpretive translation at the cost of blocking creative inspiration. Simply put, try listening less so more of you can hear a different kind of signal come through, including a thought that seems to arrive out of the blue or a question that bubbles up from the deeper unconscious well of you.

Now we can elaborate our definition of the action that precedes knowing in creative therapy. It is more accurately described as *unconsciously inspired action*. The creative therapist learns to trust what pops into the mind, including an uncommon way to talk about a common topic like problems. "I bet that problem of yours is lonely and would be happy to have a friend. Maybe we should introduce it to another problem, so it would be happier." "Would you rather work on the 'prob' or the 'lem'? Sometimes it's better to start with half the problem rather than go all the way out on a limb to deal with the whole problem." "What if we make a plea bargain with your problem? What could each of you agree to keep and eliminate?" If you must ask a client to define a problem, also insist that the definition be written and placed on either the front or back lawn. Or examine the client's shoe and ask a diagnostic question—is the issue a worn-out sole or a broken heel that never healed?

Creative therapy is both unconsciously attuned *and* empirically outcome based. This is why the creative therapist does not stop the action after every intervention or at the end of a session, pausing to inquire whether the symptom disappeared or the situation improved. Not only would this interrupt the flow, it would also make too conscious what should be left to the unconscious. The more beneficial outcome for both therapist and client is an experience that is deeply felt but cannot be easily explained, one that makes it obvious that the room is bigger and has come to life.

Creative Therapy Action Is Aided by Art, Dreams, and the Like

Gregory Bateson repeatedly warned that consciously guided action absent of correction by more unconscious wisdom is too risky a business. What "unaided consciousness (unaided by art, dreams, and the like) can never appreciate is the systemic nature of mind … mere purposeful rationality … is necessarily pathogenic and destructive of life" (Bateson, 2000/1972, pp. 145–146). Bateson's beef with the therapies of his era had more to do with their over-reliance upon purposeful rationality, something he believed would "always tend toward hate … for the … profound reason, that seeing only arcs of circuits, the individual is continually surprised and necessarily angered when his hardheaded policies return to plague the inventor" (p. 146). Bateson never called for more interpreting; he saw action and knowing as intertwined in a dialectical ladder that walked up recursive levels of process and named form (see Keeney, 1983). What he recommended was more inclusion of the unconscious so the whole "circuitry" or circularity of mind could bring its self-correcting, natural healing dynamic into play.

Bateson proposed that less consciously driven aesthetic wisdom is needed to correct and better shape pragmatic action. The art of improvisation composes such an unplanned performance that goes further into the vast unknown, rather than imposes more of the same routine. Cybernetician Heinz von Foerster elaborates—it is sensory-motor coordination and its stabilized pairing of phenomenology and action that construct a reality that includes reflections and interpretations. There is no perception separate from action and no thought distinct from circularly coupled action and perception. Put simply, thoughts are more like echoes of the action-perception loop that create them. A therapist stuck in one genre of interpretation must act differently to see and think differently, which will result in a different kind of post hoc reflection and understanding.

Making narratives or interpretations more conscious in a session (or the target of treatment) was never the kind of corrective action Bateson initially and Brad later proposed—that was nothing more than a departure from the forward steps that already had been made in the profession. The entire field of family therapy missed that Bateson only took the time during his whole career to write one positive review of a therapy book that he later did not retract. Even its main author, who had long been estranged from Bateson due to a prior conflict regarding intellectual property rights, wasn't aware of the review until Brad told him about it. The book Bateson embraced was *Change: Principles of Problem Formation and Problem Resolution.* Paul Watzlawick (1974), its senior author, had tears of joy when Brad gave him a copy of the review that had been published by Stewart Brand. As a side note, this exchange helped heal Brad's conflict with Paul Watzlawick that had arisen in the previously published controversial debates on the aesthetics and pragmatics of therapy.

Bateson was one of Brad's mentors and would have agreed, if we dare say, with Brad's later proposal that therapy become more like a performing art moved by deep wisdom, rather than a narrowly conceived event constrained by a limited range of expression with missing patterns of circularity, distanced emotion, and fractionated, partial arcs of knowing. While Bateson believed that Watzlawick and his colleagues had fallen short of achieving this, he acknowledged that they had at least taken a step closer to successfully implementing cybernetic ideas in a therapeutic context. Let us pause to fully realize how incredible it was that the body of work that Bateson praised was the exact same kind of therapy approach that postmodern collaborative and narrative therapists attacked while claiming that Bateson and his cybernetics were better exemplified by their methods of clinical work. That claim, still widely circulated today, must be carefully reexamined and courageously contested. Once again, lest it be forgotten, Bateson celebrated that Watzlawick, Weakland, and Fisch (1974) had helped liberate therapists from a century of thinking that the airing and repairing of interpretations, whether for a psychoanalytic or cultural catharsis, was the secret to making a systemic calibration (i.e. helping people change). And let us also not forget that he was equally disappointed that less of their unconscious and too much of their consciously planned strategy steered every session.

Bateson's World War II involvement in secret operations and counterintelligence (as recently released CIA documents reveal, he designed intelligence gathering in India to help maintain colonial order) left him personally ashamed of strategic action that was not held in check by greater wisdom (Price, 1998). He was thereafter always suspicious of any efforts to make a change no matter its means or ends. Bateson also admitted to Brad of rarely having personally embodied the cybernetics of which he spoke, while his descriptive accounts were more able to embody the circular action he spoke about. We can look back and see how therapists competing for a Batesonian inheritance chose to select a part or partial arc of Bateson's whole cybernetic epistemology and made themselves more alike than different—all too consciously purposeful and unaided by the performing arts, dream, healing wisdom, and the like.

Introducing the Operations of the Three-Act Performance

Part Two of the book provides transcriptions of actual sessions we have conducted with clients, though all names and identifying details have been changed to preserve anonymity. These accounts demonstrate creative therapy in practice and how it provides healing and transformation for a wide range of presenting concerns including personal crises, relationship issues, family difficulties, physical sickness, and terminal illness.

Before we proceed to the sessions, in the next chapter we will outline the basic operations involved in the production of a creative therapy session. The three-act structure hosts a specific operation for each phase that is responsible for moving a session forward: (1) Building a big room whose expansion creates the right climate for sparking and spreading change. (2) Feeding the excitement and momentum of ongoing change as the therapist skillfully sustains the expansion, infusing the session with the heat of creative expression—we call this act "getting experientially cooked by change." (3) Returning the client to the everyday with a prescription for further action that bolsters the new expanded reality that was built and transports it home with the client.

Too many sessions regrettably go nowhere and remain stuck in the opening act. If they manage to have a moment of forward movement, they quickly backslide. Or a therapist may fail to expand the room and instead shrink it, making the session more iatrogenic than healing. Creative therapy brings the skills that can help move a session forward and the discernment needed to keep track of its progress. Once a big room is constructed, the good news is that change will seem to happen spontaneously rather than purposefully. The more challenging news is that the therapist must be skillfully engaged and appropriately focused, especially in the first act where a therapeutic room is built. By the second act, beginning when the room is sufficiently altered, the interaction becomes more effortless and naturally spontaneous. This is when both therapist and client are creatively stoked as the session enthusiastically cooks. We have barely hinted how this middle phase of a creative therapy session marks it as radically different than what most therapists expect to experience in a session. We save this as a surprise that will be found in the next chapter. Finally, as the third act approaches it becomes time to wrap up the performance. The therapist now helps ready the client to reenter daily life with specific instructions, an assignment for uncommon action that helps sustain the experienced expansion and the change that was set in motion.

If you have to ask afterwards whether a session made an experiential difference, then rest assured that it probably didn't. Just like in the performing arts, the outcomes of a performance are found throughout its unfolding. Does it feel a different reality was entered where new possibilities for living are enacted rather than only posthumously imagined? Or is it chatter that goes nowhere that experientially and existentially matters? Therapy don't mean a thing if it ain't got that lean toward the big room of change. An alternative reality must be built, but this dramatically altered space must also be entered so its participants can creatively cook.

To construct a room and climate for change requires a highly skilled and multi-talented performer. If there is any hope for therapy's future, then it must become a disciplined and hard-earned art that is not dumbed down for easy workshop consumption. Therapy is as worthy of the dedicated work involved in mastering an art such as music, dance, acting, or standup comedy. An unsure therapist is easily seduced to reach for a model that can ease performance anxiety. Avoid the seduction of medicating stage fright with a therapy model serving as Modium that immobilizes unconsciously inspired action. It is time for the training wheels to come off so that therapists can grow up and learn to ride unhindered by clichés, trite lines, rigid theories, fixed models, presumptuous moralities, and canned strategies.

Creative therapy is not only about changing the client's relationship to suffering, but the therapist's own growth is also considered and valued. Carl Whitaker often surprised others, therapists and clients alike, by saying that the purpose of his sessions always included his own growth. We have encountered this same wisdom among traditional healers who don't regard a healing session as potent or effective unless they also feel transformed. Creative therapy invites practitioners to re-discover what may be the most important but rarely taught experiential compass and outcome of every session: feeling the room expand and the session come to life.

Note

1 For instance, to conduct a statistical study, variables have to be abstracted and limited to what is discrete and countable, converted into numbers and average scores suitable for computation, and plugged into a formula that generates a probability statement. The results are then only useable to negate rather than support a hypothesis that is itself already framed in a language that has no resemblance to the performance it claims to objectively evaluate. This long chain of transformed abstractions and mathematical operations requires so many leaps of faith that the investigator and therapist can easily forget what is being analyzed, confusing a statistical number with the original experience. Astonishingly, statistical outcome studies are actually the least empirical, the most hypothetical, and never a wise source of information for choosing the next course of therapeutic action.

3

THE PRACTICAL OPERATIONS OF A CREATIVE THERAPY SESSION

Every creative therapy session provides liberation from small and impoverished experiential containment via constructing and then entering a "big room" where a broader range of more resourceful, life-altering experience awaits. The sought contextual expansion is set in motion by introducing an unexpected out-of-the-box topic or responding to a client's familiar spiel in a benevolently surprising, habit-tripping, and mind-opening manner. What is addressed and how it is expressed generate an atmosphere of spontaneous creative improvisation that results in a custom-made session that is more like a new genre of theater than ordinary clinical treatment. The creative therapist's conduct readily shifts to effectively fit and flexibly alter each particular situation, rather than imposes a cliché routine of predetermined questions, prefabricated scripts, and rehashed interventions.

A creative therapy session offers a special kind of transformative experience that exudes exhilarating emotion, novel invention, and the tacit or explicit awareness of becoming a more vital part of the whole of life. The means of evoking such excitement, originality, and epiphany cannot be reduced or standardized without rendering it trivial and absent of one of its most essential qualities—*feeling* more creatively alive. This work is an art that evokes the resourceful and often mysterious treasure that lies beyond the calipers of human measure.

Creative therapy defines health as the condition of wholeness that healing aims to recover. As Wendell Berry (1997, p. 103) elaborates: "The word *health* belongs to a family of words, a listing of which will suggest how far the consideration of health must carry us: *heal, whole, wholesome, hale, hallow, holy.*" Creative therapy stands ready to address this whole continuum, starting with healing that resets any fractionated part of a person's life back into a more encompassing wholeness. It continues on until a client's life is well situated amidst an experiential space so vast that there is room for all manner of benevolent surprises to arrive from renewed elation to revitalized purpose and even an encounter with hallowed mystery. To accomplish this, creative therapy uses three main operations that lead a session through three phases or theater-like acts that will be discussed in this chapter: (1) the beginning act builds a big room; (2) the middle act is where all participants experience being cooked by change; and (3) the third and final act prepares the client for a return to the everyday with a prescription for action. This basic structure allows for an endless variety of metaphors, themes of action, and experiences to arise that are unique to every session, making creative therapy an exciting, improvisational journey that awakens, enchants, and deeply touches both practitioners and clients.

Act One: Building a Big Room

A session cannot take flight unless the therapist skillfully discerns, emphasizes, connects, and builds up metaphors and themes that widen the scope of action, conversation, imagination, and expectation. This first practical operation of creative therapy is what we call "building a big room," the nature of which is more formally described and specifically outlined by the analytical method of "Recursive Frame Analysis" (RFA) (H. Keeney, B. Keeney, & Chenail, 2015). Whether the client initially offers a specific complaint, ambiguous problem definition, clear future goal, unclear historical reference, testimony of success, list of accomplishments, tangential remark, strange metaphor, incomprehensible comment, or silence, the creative therapist does not assess either the communication or the communicant. From the first moment of a session, a revolutionary act takes place that marks the session as different from that provided by most helping professionals. The creative therapist does not utter a single word that suggests the need for a diagnosis in order to later select a corresponding intervention. All forms of diagnosis, whether psychiatric, psychological, philosophical, or spiritual in origin, arise from the same epistemology that assumes understanding the cause or nature of problematic experience is first required in order to later bring about change, and that the same method of intervention should then be applied to every client belonging to a particular category of classification. Instead, the creative therapist finds or creates an opening to another pathway that leads to either forgotten or yet to be discovered resources, wisdom, wonder, surprise, and mystery.

For instance, consider a session where a client immediately starts talking about their symptom, saying something like, "I can't stop feeling anxious. Even thinking about what I might try next to fix it makes me anxious." Here a creative therapist can immediately intervene and hold up her hand like a traffic cop stopping traffic, stand up and walk to the thermostat on the wall and reply, "Excuse me, what temperature do you prefer for the room? Do you like it more on the cool side or more on the warm side? Are you comfortable now or should I turn the thermostat up or down?" No matter what the client says, the next response continues with the temperature theme rather than rejoins the client's diagnostic discourse. "Do you find that the people you are close to prefer the same temperature as you or are they climatically different?" If the discussion of temperature is kept more interesting and engaging than a rehash of the same old same old problem talk, then the session might lead to trying out some experiments with temperature—hot mornings, cold afternoons, lukewarm sundowners, and cooler sunrises, or any other innovative variation that arises. Along these lines, the client might be encouraged to purchase a pocket fan to be used whenever the emotional climate is in need of a change. Here the client's rising and falling anxiety is transformed into thermal variety—bringing more degrees of experience with its diverse temperature settings. The same can be imagined for a client talking about depression. In that case, a tropical depression might arrive as the meteorological metaphor that leads to some altered therapeutic rainmaking.

Creative therapy ignores whatever has the presumptuous know-it-all smell of psychology, psychiatry, medicine, science, religion, New Age spirituality, self-help paradigms, or any form of explanation-based remedial treatment no matter what cloak it wears. We prefer to never know what will happen in a session, especially with regard to what will be said or done. Now consider a different client from the one above who instead of presenting an anxious concern arrives with boastful testimonies of accomplishment and endless tales of power, asking for consultation that will promote more personal advancement. Just like the creative therapist's response to a client over-saturated in problem talk, the aim is to introduce any kind of outside-the-box difference that will bring more diverse considerations to the conversation. "Thanks for showing your merit badges. Now where's your list of defeats, false turns, and total screw-ups? No one climbs to ecstasy without also wallowing in some agony. Or are you the first clean and lean success machine I have had the privilege to meet?" Another creative therapist might say: "Great, I've been waiting for someone with your talent to help me out with another case. I have a client who climbed Mount Everest and always makes sure everyone knows it was 29,029 feet or 8,840 meters high, but no matter how hard he tries to remember, he can never recall the altitude of the town where he lives. It shouldn't be a concern, but he's afraid he'll start forgetting other things about himself. What should I advise him?"

The focus of creative therapy is strictly on the journey that moves from a small room to a big room that can host a transformed relationship to both the lowest lows and highest heights. If there is any "assessment" made at the beginning of a session, it is limited to evaluating how much room there is for divergent experience. The creative therapist develops a knack for sensing shrunken contexts and skillfully avoids reinforcing or feeding any talk that either maintains or further shrinks the room that currently houses the client's experience. As the context of a session expands, interest in any search for a solution, fix, cure, trophy, pot of gold, or special badge of honor recedes as more captivating, heart-warming, and soul-searching adventures emerge. Whether a client is trying to escape what ails them or find the Holy Grail, the creative therapist avoids any form of strategic psychological combat with suffering and never cons others with false promises of an easy or cheesy walk to fame. No matter the opening gambit, immediately head toward the larger stage that hosts more significant and far-reaching transformation. Here anything from an obvious benefit to an unfathomed impossibility is given enough space to find or invent its place.

From the start, each session avoids professional jargon that contributes to additional shrinkage of the situation through labeling. We agree with Federico Fellini's suggestion that "labels should go on suitcases, and nothing else" (in Barron, et al., 1977, p. 33). We regard psychiatric nomenclature, pop psychology typologies, and spiritual taxonomies as equally small and restrictive. In order to "begin at the end" with immediate change-oriented action, a therapist must follow the Zen master's advice to drop all stories and categories. Despite clients' sincere requests for change, they can be just as attached to their preferred explanations and psychological labels as a beginning student of Zen. Like a Zen roshi, a creative therapist acts to benevolently mess with every sticky label and over-told fable, clearing the table for experience that surpasses categorical understanding.

We once had a client say to us, "I'm depressed and don't tell me I'm not because I am." Our response was: "We're not that interested in discussing whether or not you are depressed or whether someone gave you that label. We are more interested in how many different ways you can spell the word 'depression.' Here's a pen and some paper. Please spell it out for us and then allow us to carefully examine your handwriting as you misspell the word three times. Perhaps you will add four more s's to make it 'depresssssion,' or double the e's to make it 'deepreesion,' or change that 'tion' to 'shun' so it is 'depress-shun.' Go ahead and we will observe how you spell and misspell the word. One more thing, you may have heard that sometimes people think they are under a magical spell that they can't seem to break. We are not those people. We prefer thinking of spelling and misspelling while appreciating the charm of each."

The importance of expanding the contextual space that holds suffering is underscored in the Zen parable where a teacher asks his student to compare how salt tastes when it is dissolved in a small glass versus a large lake. The former tastes bitter rather than fresh because the container is too small. The suffering of life is akin to this salt; how it is experienced is determined by the size of the room within which it is held. In creative therapy the bitterness of a small glass solvent is altered, perhaps made bittersweet or more complexly seasoned when poured into a larger container's solution, now experienced as a fresh and rejuvenating tonic. Whether life brings victory or defeat, a bigger container allows for a tastier and livelier blend.

Frozen and solidified suffering thaws and dissolves when there is ample room for other kinds of experience that were formally excluded or left unnoticed. In other words, the inevitable suffering of life is blended and vindicated as part of the whole rather than mended and eradicated to serve a symptom-free psychological fantasy whose cost is too often the reduction or absence of creative vitality, greater resiliency, and aesthetic satisfaction. A well-seasoned life awakens the desire to tinker, experiment, explore, and play, inviting further creative involvement with whatever the universe sets on stage. When a creative therapy performance stretches toward richer experiential diversity, it embraces the practical wisdom that holds all the seasons of life including tragedy and comedy, as well as agony and ecstasy, while driving with the creative license to shift, alter, and change anything ripe for transformation.

The longer a therapist remains inside the same small room initially introduced by a client, the more difficult it is to exit. Clients essentially come to a session prepared to say in some kind of coded or camouflaged way, "I'm stuck and unable to stretch and move inside this small bottle—I can't escape it." We come prepared to respond, "You are like a model ship placed inside a bottle, but you and the bottle are actually floating and bobbing on an immense sea. Let's uncork the bottle, pour you out, reopen your sails, and see where the wind takes you." The sooner the horizon is expanded, the more possible a voyage on the vast blue sea becomes. If needed, a creative therapist can even tell a client a Zen-riddled parable as a means of keeping the session on course. But never do so unless the sail and window are open, so the wind can blow the story away when its performance is over. Make sure the dramatic action sails ahead of the tale so the voyage finds its way over the *rain* and the *bow* (rain: the weather change that opens seeds and nurtures growth; bow: the most forward part of the boat, the ribbon that puts the final touch on a gift, and what a performer does after a stunning performance).

The focus and locus of creative therapy is the whole container, existential room, space, contextual frame, matrix, or ecology that holds a client's everyday life rather than any isolated part or participant within it. Aim to make room for what lies beyond what the client formerly presumed was attainable, realizable, sensible, logical, and believable, moving them outside their familiar narrow surroundings into the broader sphere and atmosphere of life's ongoing creation with all its change, transformation, and growth. Here they find more than the assignment of a menial nametag and its induced nightmare of being reduced to the causality of molecule, neuron, endocrine drip, bad childhood trip, or any other fantasized fault, bitter salt, lion's den, or pathogen. A small room binds you to misery while a big room places you, and life's intermittent misery, inside mystery. We even once asked a client in a session when it was time to shift gears, "Shall we wallow in misery or take a break and find some mystery?"

Clients require a therapist who is change-worthy, that is, more improvisationally and resourcefully responsive to each moment as a session unfolds. The wisdom proverb, "Physician, heal thyself," must be taken further to prescribe, "Therapist, change thyself" in order to assure steadfast expansion of the whole situation. We once supervised a trainee from behind a one-way mirror and it was obvious that the session was not going anywhere. We rang the telephone in the treatment room, as is often done in this kind of live supervision, but we asked to speak to the client and not the therapist. "Here's the situation," we said to the client. "We need to figure out how to wake up your therapist. When she gets therapeutically awakened, you won't believe how the session will change. You are in for a surprise when this takes place. Here's our recommendation: consider asking her whether she wants to discuss your *shoestrings*. Then take off one shoe, remove the shoestring, and place it on the empty chair next to you. Let's see what she does with that surprise. We will call again if that's all right with you. Thank you. Go ahead and make this happen." The interactions of this session creatively came to life when the therapist became the client and the client became the co-therapist with the supervisor. When the whole system of interaction is the client, any member of the interaction can be the recipient or the agent of change.

During a different session with another trainee, we rang the phone and told the therapist to take a break and come out for a consultation. We told him that we were going to enter the room for a chat with the client who was an older woman worried about whether her life had been a success or a failure. We went into the room as he now observed the action. Our words to the client: "We notice that you are a caring mother and grandmother who has raised many children. May we ask you to use some of that skill to help us develop and grow this young therapist? We noticed how kind you are with him and we want you to know that he is very nervous about doing a good job in front of us. Could you do something to help him feel more confident about being able to help you in this session? You could start by saying, 'I think I'm ready to make a little change.' Do you think it would be better for me to start grandmothering other people outside my family relations or keep my skills locked up inside the home?" Not only did the interaction that ensued immediately change the session, it altered the way the client's home life. Finally, one year later we hired her as a clinical consultant to assure that we had more access to the wisdom voice of a grandmother whenever it was needed.

Creative therapy's initial operation of room expansion always includes more social inclusion because the client is never conceived as an isolated individual. Like pioneer family therapist, Carl Whitaker,[1] we boldly regard the notion of a psychologically defined "individual"—a personality *in vitro*—as an illusory mirage that obscures awareness of the surrounding human ecology. A whole system of relations rather than an epidermal outline or heap of atoms walks through the session door. This system minimally includes the helped and the helper(s) as well as the whole social relational fabric of which they are a part. Enlarge the room to make space for a herd of others that may include family, friends, colleagues, community, and even imaginary characters from Shakespeare to Mother Mary and Father Time. Both client *and* therapist must together, through their interaction, break through the walls of solitary confinement and step into a more spacious reality that serves transforming everyone participating in a session and those who will be affected afterwards.

"I don't want my family coming to the session," said a client on the phone. We answered, "They are already on their way." The client again protested, "May I come alone for the first session?" We compromised, "Only if we can include a conference call with the rest of your folks or text them ongoing reports." We once had another client agree to see us in our car that was parked in the clinic parking lot as long as his mother sat in a car next to us. We rolled down the windows and he was able to keep her separate while we could also include her in the session—an intervention that enacted a family change. These are examples of how family therapists used to talk—a form of change-oriented rhetoric that is slipping away as contemporary family therapists see more individuals and fewer families. The unfortunate result is there is more talk with individuals *about* their relationships and less skill in working with the whole family during its interaction.

Creative therapy also regards terms like "consciousness," "individuation," "self-actualization," and "self-realization" as straying too far from big room metaphors. They promote blindness to the way life resides in the interstitiality or "in-betweenness" of an ecosystem rather than a biological shell. Human beings are no exception to ecological rule—we experientially exist and subsist as an inseparable part of all our relations, whether we consciously notice or not. This bigness of life—its whole ecology—can only be experienced in a big room. When systemic or relational themes are discussed in a small theoretical chamber rather than enacted in a vaster container, every person still remains an island. From the eco-systemic or big room perspective, the client in a creative therapy session consists of more than what meets the conventionally trained eye. As discussed in chapter two, the "client" is the room that hosts the ongoing interaction of everyone inside it. This may also include family members, or even beloved pets, from the past and present who powerfully reside inside the client's memory or imagination.

A creative therapy session requires that a therapist and client (and supervisor when present) change in relationship to one another while they are a part of an ongoing interaction. As an old African proverb advised, "If you want to go far, go together." The therapist must go further than the world of psychological rumination, the myth of individual treatment, and the limitations of solitary recovery. It takes a changing interaction to move everyone involved into the big room where change is cooking.

In summary, the beginning operation of act one is to build a big room that liberates those in attendance, escaping the impoverished living quarters they brought upon arrival. Move the client, along with the therapist and all others involved, from a small psyche bottle to a bigger-than-self space that is more inclusive of not only one's immediate relationships, but also openly embraces the broader surroundings. The mystery of higher-order change resides in the web of life where the residuals called individuals become resituated and reactivated inside interactions that reconstitute a reawakened wholeness.

The Big Room Is Built by Turning a Virtuous Wheel of Change

The most common mistake of a beginning therapist involves not taking the time or doing the construction work that make the room big enough to host the experience of profound change. A big room cannot be built with one action, an isolated behavioral sequence, a particular question, a singular solution, a one-time mention of a presumed reframe, or a hypnotic induction alone. These are all mirages of the "magic bullet" delusion whose reductionist premise is not dissimilar from offering a pill to make the client well. It takes an ongoing stream of interaction that never stops creatively improvising to build and then sustain an expansive room. This progression does not ride the lineal track of simple causality. It is circular—a virtuous circle that must constantly turn.

All human experience, whether it involves what's resourceful or troubling, is organized by the same underlying circular dynamic that we metaphorically call "the wheel of change." When this wheel spins toward a wide-open range of experience it operates a bit like a tumbleweed that gathers unexpected surprises, becoming larger and more filled with different items as it keeps on rolling. It may pick up a feather, a bone, a flower, a lost love letter, or a can of tobacco—anything that can contribute to a richer and more interesting life. However, if the tumbleweed is limited to rolling inside a small fenced-in horse corral, it can only gather what lies on that small patch of smelly ground. Like the tumbleweed, in order for the wheel of change to get rolling toward the open pasture it needs someone to help bust open the corral gates and get it moving in another direction toward a vaster space.

The direction the wheel of change turns in a session and the space it traverses are steered by whatever is emphasized in the therapeutic interaction.

Clients already come to therapy with a wheel that is spinning in a vicious direction, keeping them in an existentially constricted corral. Impoverished experience is unintentionally maintained when therapists offer the same kind of talk and action that the client is steeped in. The wheel then gains momentum in the direction that shrinks the space as it gathers more of the same kind of content inside it, resulting in even less room for mobilizing an escape.

The direction the wheel of change turns[2] determines whether the room expands or shrinks. Building a big room uses the same circular dynamic that shrinks a room but reverses the wheel's direction by underscoring and feeding whatever metaphors, themes, and action can take a session somewhere new and more interesting—more therapeutically untypical and not previously expected. For example, if a client asks, "Can you help me, doc?" A creative therapy outlaw who refuses to be fenced in by a model is freer to reply, "I was hoping you'd help me change the way I usually answer such a question." Another creative therapist might choose to respond with, "Why don't we assume you'll never change and then discuss how you can do something else with your life other than try to find a solution?" A creative therapist can always tap into the family system to widen the scope of exploration: "What would your mother definitely *not* say about your situation?" Or "What if an older brother you never knew you had suddenly arrived and answered your question?" For those more absurdly daring, hand out an artistically designed card that has these words carefully handwritten on it: "Remember what the wise old red tomato from Mesopotamia once inscribed with a twinkle in its stem, 'Being read doesn't mean you can write a wrong.'" If a more direct Ericksonian twist is preferred, then consider: "I can only help you if you convince my unconscious that it should come up with some help that is worth the effort." Or hand the client a penny, nickel, or dime and seriously ask, "How can we exchange this for some better felt change?" And finally, go ahead and reach for the highest bar: "Do you prefer your session shaken or stirred?"

In each of the above examples, the therapist interrupts the momentum of a viciously turning wheel and gives it an initial push in a more creative direction. There is no imposition of a therapy model that fences everyone in. Clients who encounter therapists who work with a model end up in a duel between corrals—the client's fenced-in room faces the therapist's fenced-in room and the two go at it. Both need liberation and a ride on the change range. Sometimes therapists fear they aren't creative enough to leave their model, but this is because the model has made them act like a tumbleweed that is only allowed to roll around on a tiny patch of ground, cut off from all the treasure found underneath a vaster sky. On the wide-open range a therapist may spontaneously burst into music, singing along with Roy Rogers and Dale Evans: "Here on the range I belong, drifting along with the tumbling tumbleweeds." More importantly, therapists are surprised to see how naturally creative they can be after the corral is left for a broader adventure. The range that is the creative therapist's home is wide and stretches across a more expansive horizon that includes the unconscious, as well as dreams and songs that inspire. With all these resources in tow a creative therapist is better equipped to follow the scent of a different kind of trail, discerning more opportunities to get the wheel turning in a virtuous direction that follows a client's laugh, surprise, double take, irrational outburst, unruliness, passion, and emotional elation while giving less attention to the habituated head nod of minimal participation in a conversation.

Even nonsense talk can move the wheel in a virtuous direction and bring more life to a session, and that includes offering absurd diagnoses. For example, we have diagnosed clients with "creative constipation," "broken funny bones," "repressed accessories," "incomplete depression," "imperfect anxiety," "inoperable stubbornness," "chronic embarrassment avoidance," "reverse amnesia that forgets the future," "the odd couple syndrome," "faulty bedroom grammar," "closet shock stock," "leaving-home jitters," "philosophical hysteria," "allergy to foreign words," "kitchen malpractice," "addiction to boring explanations," "bargain basement problem," "higher ordeal," "undeveloped absurds," "culturally inappropriate mojo," "irritable vowel syndrome," "uncontrollable dia-lie-a," "fable inflation," "existential transport issues," "chronic sonic aversions," "outgrown trance," "psychotic recreation selection," "dictionary deprivation," "bed meta-ing," "spiritual heart burn," and "ghost trouble" to name a few from our handbook of alternative labels.

In order for the wheel of change to move in a virtuous direction, a therapist cannot simply change the subject of conversation from so-called "negative" to "positive" topics. This is the naïve error of "positive thinking" that excludes what it dislikes while shrinking rather than extending the existential space. The valence matters less than creating more room that is able to include all the plusses and minuses. Whereas a constantly complaining client might need to look up, a boasting client can equally benefit from looking down—each action makes more room for diverse experience. For example, we once invited a burned-out solution-focused therapist to offer a "catastrophe question" to the next client: "What's the worst catastrophe you could imagine happening in the next two minutes? Make sure it would be interesting enough to make the front page of *The New York Times*. How about a meteor shower that takes place *inside* the room? Or what if your guardian angel walked through the wall and angrily announced that you aren't providing anything interesting enough to guard?" The fine line between miracles and catastrophes is analogous to the thin separation between solutions and problems—each side of any opposite is linked to the other. To make a difference that makes a creative difference, avoid highlighting one side of a distinction at the expense of the other. Instead, play with the line—bend it, wiggle it, or turn it into an Ouroborean circle.

The more often therapists take a cybernetic walkabout outside the box of therapy, the more they become tumbleweeds full of interesting objects, creative ideas, unusual questions, and remarkable dreams that are ready to pop up when needed in their sessions. In our sessions we have discussed ambivalent angels, friendly demons, unknown critters, skipping stones, broken branches, spooky tones, and invisible relations. And we have asked odd questions such as: "What grammatically misplaced apostrophe might accidentally precipitate a calamity? Don't think about it, just draw an apostrophe on the palm of your hand and wonder whether it might cause a most unfortunate spelling." Apostrophes, catastrophes, and miracles are equally capable of generating a "difference." In creative therapy, anything can happen as long as the therapist is able to discern from one moment to the next which way the wheel of change is moving, ready to continue on or alter the course that keeps a session on track toward a bigger room.

It takes tremendous skill to get the wheel of change smoothly turning toward a more inclusive space, a broader ecology, and eventually a whole alternative reality. It requires the immediate outcome-based orientation discussed in chapter two, as well as the participation of the therapist's creative unconscious that is better equipped to steer the wheel. After each step taken toward expansion, it is natural for the client to interject former habituated concerns that don't yet readily seem to fit into the room that is in formation. How the creative therapist responds will determine whether there is a return to the previous small container or whether that former reality can be placed inside the room under construction.

For example, if a therapist invites creative exploration of formerly forgotten moments of bliss, "repressed memories of joy," or creatively reinvented pasts, the conversation may discuss previous wonder-full vacations, favorite toys, remarkable episodes of hilarity, unexplainable magical moments from the client's childhood, or imaginary friends and relatives that were invented in the past or created now in the session. Should a client throw in some bitter salt from the past, it doesn't have to immediately shift the focus, derail the momentum, and shrink the room again by turning the wheel back in a vicious direction. Instead, a therapist can appear surprised and quickly respond with a statement like, "There are so many things we forget from the past, aren't there?" Then immediately shift gears, while staying within the same general class of forgotten memories without emphasizing the formerly specified one: "Do you remember the first time you tasted a lemon or a spoonful of honey? What was the first joke you ever heard? How about the second joke? Do remember your earliest bedtime story or lullaby? How about your initiatory jump over a rope?" However, if a client is only able to boast, exaggerate, or accentuate the positive, then make room to ask about the first finger splinter, foot blister, or bloody nose. Or discuss the most interesting former embarrassment or missed opportunity. Whether the client's talk is missing sweet or sour experience, the room is made larger by adding different kinds of forgotten memories, neither ignoring any of them nor inflating any particular type to become a mini-container that has no room for other kinds of unremembered experience.

The creative therapist never forgets that each session enacts some variation of the old Zen water treatment: when the container that holds suffering is small like a glass, life tastes bitter; however, if the container is as big as the sea, then bitter experiences are free to mix, mingle, and transform. The vast sea also invites getting on board a ship whose journey has no need to fuss about a glass, drink, or taste. In other words, serve more seas than glasses to clients who arrive thirstier for change than another bitter reminder that they are living in the wrong container. When the therapist successfully enables the inclusion of small room experience inside a freshly expanded space, it enriches the new reality, contributes to expansion, and further turns the virtuous wheel of change. Rather than fight or ignore the reappearance of a former habit, give it a new habitat and resituate it as a part of a newly emerging big room.

The beginning act of a session is like a contest between small and big rooms. When the therapist expands the room, it automatically deflates the parts of a client's experience that formerly took up so much space that they felt like the whole room. Take whatever clients assume is the whole container of their life and make it a part of something larger. Expect that any forward step toward the big room may result in the client pointing to or taking a step back into a former small room. Rather than regress with them, create an unexpected incorporation where former small room experience is brought even more fully inside the emerging big room. Conflicts, problems, and suffering are not banned from the big room; they are invited, but in a way that puts them inside a vaster existential space. They then are experienced as less dominating, more resourcefully involved, and better dissolved within the greater phenomenal diversity of a whole big room that exudes rather than excludes creative change.

Act Two: Getting Experientially Cooked by Change

The operations of act one never cease as the therapist continuously works throughout the session to build and maintain presence inside a big room. After enough space has been built, however, a tipping point takes place that clearly indicates that act two has begun. As the wheel of change gains momentum and turns more effortlessly, the therapist feels the room increasingly expand, bringing creative energy along with it. The session starts to rock and sway between the small room where the session began and the big room under construction, creating a fulcrum between act one and act two. At some point the session fully tips toward the newly constructed reality. The primary operation of act two then kicks in as the therapist helps circulate the feeling of change in the atmosphere, drawing upon a wider range of expression and emotion.

In past discussions of creative therapy, we described the three acts of a session solely in terms of how their progression builds an ever-expanding therapeutic reality. Act two was described as straddling a fulcrum that teeter-totters between the initial diminished space and the sought transition to a big room. The interaction rocks back and forth until it moves fully inside the new expanded room. This transition marks the start of the third and final act in which the goal of full occupancy in an alternative therapeutic reality is reached. Inside act three an intervention is given that helps the client remain within that reality and maintain the momentum of change after the session ends.

We previously were not yet ready to disclose the next operation of creative therapy—our exposition was still a work in progress. While our previous discussions exclusively emphasized the construction of a big room over the course of all three acts, what we didn't say is that there is another operation that comes into play in the second act that further feeds and empowers the process of expansion and its accompanying changes. When the session crosses the tipping point and act two commences, there is a natural awakening of creative excitement that inspires a wider range of expression. This heightened emotion is expressed by the therapist and felt by everyone in the room. As increased expansion, intensified emotional excitement, and spontaneous expression are coordinated, the room comes alive in a noticeable way as everyone is experientially cooked by all the changing that is taking place.

During the second act of a session, the creative therapist leaves the familiar territory of western psychotherapy and finds what has been critically missing over all the years since Freud first reported Irma's injection dream in Vienna and gave birth to the much younger folk healing tradition of psychotherapy. Before Freud's first patient reclined and even before the Viennese danced their first waltz, many healing traditions around the globe had discovered a means of igniting the kind of change that experientially transforms lives—something now openly welcomed and embraced in a creative therapy session. The creative therapist, like a traditional healer, is attuned to what most social science and medical models will not allow in their ideation or performance space. It is an operation—the second main operation of creative therapy—that is more difficult to define because it is not a matter of cognition, but a creative kind of ignition that is energetically felt when it appears. Many performing artists know it but cannot explain it and are unsure what to name it. It is sometimes simply called "the creative life force" that inspires, moves, and guides the performer, aesthetically distinguishing a performance as an art rather than an enactment of rote technique.

This impossible-to-measure and unseen force, enthusiastically welcomed by traditional healers and performing artists and fiercely excluded by reductionist social science practitioners, is equivalent to the Kalahari Bushman healer's *n/om*, the Japanese seiki jutsu master's *seiki*, the sanctified church goer's *holy spirit*, and what Dr. Robert Fulford, the former renowned osteopathic healer, simply called the *universal life force*. We refer to it as both the creative life force and the "ecstatic pulse" because is felt as a heightened emotion *and* a tingling current or vibrating pulse in the body. This somatic kinesthetic experience is the old school healing means of discerning whether a session is dead or alive. The creative life force is as strong as the room is big, and it is missed or dismissed in most psychotherapy sessions because students are never told about it when they receive their education. To experience what healers and creative therapists most exalt, leave the sensory memory of a bland clinic behind and learn to experience the pulse of a big room. When the vibrant buzz and heightened emotion of the creative life force are missing in a session, everyone feels lifeless and exhausted. But when the fuse of change is lit and the creative muse comes to life, no one wants the session to end.

Creative therapists follow the same tracks of traditional ecstatic healers whose somatic inner excitement guides and shapes the action. It is like having a special kind of inner Geiger counter that lets a therapist know how big the room is and how smoothly the wheel is virtuously turning. We respectfully acknowledge that this somatic experience remains foreign to those who have not experienced it. However, when this experience is established as a new inner reference point, the creative therapist is better equipped to construct a big room, sustain it, and help it crackle with inspiration. The performance goal is to go beyond any lifeless conversation about a fixit, trauma, mama, papa, stuck state, or frozen fate. Instead, creative therapy steps into the big room where change is pulsing, energizing, exciting, creating, expanding, and cooking—the second operation of creative therapy that comes to life in act two of a session.

One of the basic tenets of traditional healing is that the construction of a big room is itself an extraordinary act of change—it brings newborn vitality as it resets and realigns everyone to be touched by unexpected experience. In this space human beings are more changeable—there is greater room for unconscious wisdom, wild imagination, and creatively inventive expression to come through. While both the operations of room expansion and life force awakening are co-present from the start of a session, the second operation does not fully kick in until the room is big enough to feel it rise to primary importance. Once the session is full of the energy and freshly awakened emotion of creative change, a therapist is more authentically able to run around the room, drop a feather, squirt a clown's flower, pull out a shoestring, sing to a glass of water, sit on a map, pretend to dance on eggshells, howl like a wolf, or listen to seashells—all of which we have done and more. We even gave a couple a pair of "shell-phones" from the sea so they could have a different kind of cellular communication.

If a client comes to us hoping to experience "ecstatic healing" instead of "therapy," we are open and ready to voice a mantra, offer a prayer, sing a sacred song, or ceremonially dance, but only if the time, space, and feeling are right. The creative therapist only conducts such action on a big room stage when the whole atmosphere is favorable enough to inspire it. Even cursing can be as nourishing as praying when the context is right, just as a blessing can become a curse when given in the wrong kind of room. Rather than presumptuously exalt or ban any particular action, including what is presumed to be therapeutic or non-therapeutic, learn to build a big room and be guided by the pulse of the creative life force so that whatever serves change can freely come forth when the moment is right.

Each creative therapy session searches for the wakeup zap, the exuberant tap, and the rhyming rap while minimizing or ignoring whatever is deadly still, sounds discordantly shrill, and feels emotionally chilled. This hunt for the creative life force begins in act one when it is dormant, hidden, or asleep. The therapist can sense, both with their body and their deeper unconscious, that the session has not yet come to life, and this is in part what helps the therapist discern what to feed and what to ignore, that is, which metaphors and themes expand the room and which ones shrink it. Once the room is big enough and the wheel of change has enough momentum, the creative life force fully wakes up and becomes the dominant operation and main star of act two. There is a symbiotic relationship between room expansion and life force awakening—one is not possible without the other. Constructing a big room and creatively cooking inside it are as much about wisely ignoring, deconstructing, and teasing away whatever leads people astray as they are about giving the most attention and celebration to any unexpected metaphor, 'pataphysical pataphor, movement, rhythm, tone, or emotion that turns the wheel of change. Passive discussion and lifeless reflection result in a session that goes nowhere meaningful and is unable to noticeably change a life. For a session to advance to act two and experientially cook, the therapist must physically, emotionally, and expressively come to life, so the client can do the same.

Circulating the Ecstatic Pulse

When the creative life force wakes up in act two, it immediately inspires the widening of the therapist's range of expression to match the emotional tenor and climate of the room. More rhythm and melodic tone enter the therapist's speech, along with a noticeable vibration in the voice. Natural, spontaneous movement kicks in as well, usually involving gentle rocking and swaying. Finally, tactile contact with the client may take place through hand-to-hand contact. This brings a new experience to therapy, a handshake that hosts a trembling ideomotor movement. This handheld vibration, along with the vocalized vibration of melodic speech that may even lead to singing, provides a different means of conveying and circulating the ecstatic pulse that awakens in the middle act of a creative therapy session. Rather than ignore or dampen the felt presence of the creative life force, creative therapy welcomes its circulation in the room.

The handshake that conveys ideomotor trembling is one of the most unique and least expected contributions of creative therapy. This tactile contact and kinesthetic interaction are only offered when a therapist feels sufficiently ready, inspired, and comfortable with its introduction. Since it involves ideomotor movement rather than purposefully orchestrated motion, the therapist never knows beforehand whether it will be performed. When the ecstatic pulse is felt strongly enough, the therapist reaches for the client's hand with a choreographed motion similar to an everyday handshake. With the client's permission, the therapist and client proceed with a handshake that enables ideomotor movement to be shared as it is mutually held.

While a client's hand is held, the vibration in the therapist's body registers the extent to which the room has expanded and the extent to which its creative energy has intensified— the vital signs of the transformative process. There is no need to keep this a secret from the client. "Do you feel that tremble? That's the pulse of the session. Now you're really cooking. Great, let's allow change to work on you." Or more indirectly: "That's right, let the back and forth movement itself handle whatever needs to be mixed inside of you. Let the oscillation of this vibration shake up all the parts of you. As all the lefts and the rights of you, the ups and downs of you, the formerly resolved and the still unresolved aspects of you, and all the this's and that's of you come together to say 'hello' to one another, encourage them to work together to come up with a new blend of you." There is also no need to say a thing unless inspired to, and instead, just let the shared movement enact whatever's felt, allowing it to speak louder than words.

Though not all sessions reach the point where a trembling handshake is made, each and every session does become altered enough to bring a noticeable rhythmic pulse and a vibrant melodic tone to the therapist's voice. When a session begins to creatively cook, the therapist's speech becomes more poetically rendered, rhythmically metered, and musically toned. It is this altered expression of the therapist that indicates that the middle act of creative therapy is in play. The bigger the room, the more a creative therapist experiences the strength of the session's ecstatic pulse, that is, the degree to which change is alive, expanding, and cooking the session.

During the middle act, more emotion and motion come to life in a noticeably energized room. Everyone feels touched and afterwards ready to reenter the world in a different way. With the ecstatic pulse as a benchmark, therapy navigates new and unexplored territory for the helping professions—making it more able to extend the longitude, raise the latitude, and improve the attitude about bringing on the heat that cooks the experience of change.

The ecstatic pulse can also be amplified and shared through music. In our sessions, when things are ready to cook Brad heads to the piano and provides musical accompaniment to whatever is said, now voiced more melodically. A Broadway song may be played or any other kind of music, with improvised new lyrics designed for the client based on the metaphors and themes that arose in the session. In this therapeutic cabaret, the client more deeply feels the transformation that has been set in motion. The stronger the emotion, the more the unconscious is receptive and involved. It is one thing to utter a therapeutic line to a client with the typical timbre and tone, but it is an entirely different experience to sing it to the score of *Oklahoma*, *West Side Story*, or *Camelot*. Sometimes only the blues will do, and other times the therapist is best accompanied by Beethoven. Stephen Sondheim can also motivate and activate the kind of word play that delivers some interesting news, whether it's "a funny thing happened on the way to the forum" or a reminder to "merrily roll along" so "not a day goes go by" without the need to remember that "anyone can whistle."

If you wish, you may consider this as a new kind of musically induced and emotionally fueled trance that supplements, enhances, deepens, and intensifies the kinetic trance (Akstein, 1992) already taking place through trembling hands or a swaying body. This kind of kinetic, hypnotic, ecstatic, theatrical, and musical cooking is something new to both therapy and the performing arts. Too often music therapy, dance therapy, and art therapy contextualize the arts inside the therapy room where psychological or self-help diagnosis and interpretation rein. In creative therapy, the therapy room is ejected so the performance goes higher and higher, landing in the theater and/or the healing ceremonies of old, or hybrids and new genres not yet categorized.

Don't expect a session to always involve song, dance, trembling handshakes, ceremonial ritual, or mystical metaphor. Also remember that the mere mention of a word the therapist presumes to be full of mystery or wonder is not enough to make a space vast. As the case examples in this book will show, big room metaphors are different from one client and session to the next and need to emerge from the interaction itself. Again, creative therapy aims to expand the performance stage, not impose a particular form. Some sessions will seem less creatively charged or ecstatically alive than others—this is natural. Rushing to enact any fantasy of what a creative therapy session is supposed to look and sound like usually fails because the therapist failed to work inside the interaction with the client, building the right room to host such an experience. Make sure that movement toward the big room involves less knowing and more circularly virtuous flowing, accepting that a session will reach the appropriate degree of expansion that a client needs for the situational moment. What will always remain true for a creative therapy session, however, is that it comes alive and enters the second act when the therapist feels the ecstatic pulse awaken, allowing it to guide subsequent action and expansion so that a session can creatively cook.

The Creative Therapy Thermometer

Many ecstatic healing traditions have a way of talking about their transformative work that is not found in therapy. They use temperature metaphors to describe a session, calling it "hot," "warm," "cool," or "cold." The more that heightened emotion of the ecstatic jubilant kind is felt, the more that the body moves with an altered rhythm and the voice speaks in a melodically embellished tone. This "heat" is regarded by ecstatic healers as the climatic condition needed to help others heal and transform. Furthermore, the experiential outcome sought is referred to as being "cooked." This is why the middle act of creative therapy is called "getting cooked by change."

Following the practical wisdom of ecstatic healers, we created the term "spiritual thermometer" (Keeneys, 2016) to keep track of the range of experience and expression that can take place in a session. When addressing the field of psychotherapy, we apply this metaphor but alter its name to be the "creative therapy thermometer" to avoid any non-resourceful associations therapists may have with spirituality or religion. The thermometer is a practical tool that discerns the degree of heartfelt emotion, motion, rhythm, melodic tone, life force current, and ecstatic pulse both experienced and expressed in a session, with less confusion and conceptual baggage brought by other more abstract means of evaluating a performance. For example, a therapist who incorporates spiritual metaphors and "mindfulness" practices into her sessions may be operating at the same temperature as a traditional psychiatrist. On the other hand, a secular psychiatrist like Milton Erickson entered a warmer zone when he activated more poetic talk voiced with an altered tone.

We have found that traditional ecstatic healers are the least concerned with a practitioner's professed beliefs or professional title. It matters little whether a helper calls herself a therapist, counselor, coach, healer, or shaman. What matters is whether the host can make a session hot enough to cook in order to foster realignment, retuning, rebirth, deconstruction and reconstruction, mending, making whole, and all the other metaphors for transformation. "Getting cooked" is shorthand for any and all of these described outcomes as well as a reference to the second operation involved in a creative therapy session.

Along the whole spectrum of the creative therapy thermometer is found the entire range of expression a therapist may offer. Since creative therapy belongs to the house of performance, all the performing arts are welcomed from poetry to acting, drawing, sculpting, photography, juggling, singing, yodeling, auctioneering, vocal improvising, drumming, instrument playing, and dancing, to name a few. In the coldest zones of the creative therapy temperature scale reside the use of memorized treatment protocols and recitations. Somewhere between cold and hot are found the moderate temperatures where a therapist creatively thaws. This is when the therapist wakes up and exhibits more improvised, creative expression. As the temperature continues to elevate, the ecstatic pulse strengthens and is more readily shared through altered vocal tone and rhythm, tactile hand-to-hand contact, music, or movement. While this creative operation enlivens and inspires, further intense emotion of a sacred nature is required for the room to sizzle with the fervor found in an ecstatic healing context. Only in the hottest temperature is found the uncommon peak experience of healing ecstasy that brings an awe-inspiring encounter with the numinous—the classic spiritual cooking found among the Kalahari Bushmen and the Shakers of St. Vincent, among others.

For the most part creative therapy remains, like other performing arts, in the "creative melt zone" where an artist straddles cool established forms *and* warmed up creative improvisation. This temperature zone should not be regarded as less transformative or less potent than a Kalahari spiritual cook-out. As people who have experienced both, we can say that in the creative melt is found one of the most aesthetically satisfying and existentially powerful experiences of change. The sessions we present in this book emphasize this temperature range of creative expression, though some venture higher up the thermometer. Anything too hot cannot be easily depicted by a written transcription or description because its essential communication is better heard and felt, not told in the cold.

The temperature a session reaches should be determined by the interaction with the client, not a predetermined thermostat setting made by the therapist. Recall that the lineal movement of a session from small room to big room and from cool to warm is actually organized by a (cybernetic) wheel of change. If a practitioner is fully inside the wheel with a client, rather than dissociated and removed, the temperature rise and room size will be naturally regulated to best serve change. If you can't imagine singing with your clients, for example, it just means that you have not yet learned to build the kind of room in which such action comes forth naturally when the time is right for it. We invite therapists to break free from the psychotherapy profession's pre-programmed thermostat setting that reflects a bias toward cold temperature and the presumption that this is what clients prefer or is what best serves change.

With the creative therapy thermometer, a therapist can gauge whether a session room is small, frigid, and rigid or whether it is expanding, warming, and moving with creative life. Practitioners are then better informed and more ready to exit all ideas and action associated with anything other than those that turn up the temperature. We once warmed a session by asking about a grandparent's favorite flavor of ice cream and strategizing ways for a grandchild to be funnier. We turned up the thermostat in other sessions by discussing the last time a client was truly startled by a train whistle, dog bark, coyote howl, cat meow, owl hoot, trumpet toot, or ship horn. We once put three fortune cookies on the table and asked the surprised client to open each and select the most intriguing divination. In another session, we investigated the last time anyone mentioned the client's middle name. Preferring the entertainment of ventriloquism over the entrainment of somnambulism, another creative therapy session explored whether a family pet spoke at home. This question led to exploring the family's theatrically projected vocal tones. It is creatively more sizzling to ask a client to remove lint, pull a loose thread of fabric, manufacture a sneeze, or react oddly to a chilly breeze than it is to invite another replay of an explanatory freeze. Go for the big bang of transformative dynamite rather than the fizzle of annoying babble that misfires and tires. To defeat whatever is emotionally cold and existentially dead, head for the fire of change. We never know how big or heated the space will get, but if we effectively do our job, the room will expand, the temperature will rise, and the wheel of change will virtuously turn as needed.

Without exception, therapeutic heat and tingly excitement are evident in the expression of a creative therapist whenever the big room is built and entered in act two. As the wheel of change picks up momentum it sparks increased emotion and releases more of the creative life force. Again, this automatically triggers a change in the therapist's voice and manner of speech. More poetic metaphor, singsong speech, and vibratory vocalization match the excitement experienced as the ecstatic pulse's dynamic presence is more strongly felt. At this point, a creative therapy session is clearly perceived as having gone past the limits of therapy and coaching. Here the creative therapist looks like the performer and reformer of a new kind of transformative art—an invoking, provoking, evoking, deconstructing, reconstructing conductor of change that is mediated by the widest range of creative expression.

As mentioned, our sessions always have a keyboard nearby that Brad plays when the room is ready for invented-in-the-moment lyrical lines and rhymes, accompanied by music of any genre that may include atonality and noise. Hillary brings chanting, percussion, singing, spontaneous drawing, syncopated clapping, and improvised dancing. With whatever expressive gifts are at hand, a creative therapist performs with the chops they own. If you are naturally hilarious, then your sessions need to be more orthopedic and help clients find their funny bones, wherever they may be hiding.

One of the other signatures of our creative therapy sessions takes place when Hillary quickly sketches a drawing of a theme that has emerged during a session. It can be a serious symbol, a hilarious cartoon, an illustrated summary of the prescription, or an unexpected image that evokes what was felt. She has drawn boats, animals, imaginary scenes, family crests, zany maps, otherworldly flowers, bees and hives, and anything that strikes her creative fancy during the session. When clients accept a drawing made during the creative heat of a session, an image or symbol of the room that was built and the change that was set in motion during the hour physically goes home with them.

Once we supervised a therapist working with a couple in a university clinic in Louisiana. A boost of change was needed so we walked into the room and invited the couple to walk over and take a look at a large painting that was hanging on the clinic wall. After a few minutes of discussion about the painting (in which we made both touching and humorous connections between its contents and the couple's situation), we surprised them by taking it off the wall and advising the couple to take it home and hang it up for a week. Both the therapist and the couple went into a cataleptic-like trance, totally surprised and shocked by what was occurring. Then, upon recognizing the unexpected absurdity of the moment, everyone broke into wild laughter and the couple became the most excited we'd ever seen them. They proudly and enthusiastically walked out with a big painting to temporarily hang on their living room wall. We have done the same with clients we saw in our home, sometimes letting them keep a painting after hearing the changes it awakened so that it could continue to redecorate their lives when the therapy had ended.

The degree of change fostered by a creative therapy session is reflected in what can be seen, heard, and felt in the expression of the therapist. As we have suggested over the years, it is past due for the transformative arts to depart from social science and medical science and instead head to the open stage of the performing arts where there is more room to creatively act and dynamically express. The original healers were singers, dancers, drummers, musicians, actors, ceremonialists, priests, clowns, artists, and all the other names for creative performers that aimed to help liberate diminished existence. The contemporary helping professions have cut themselves off from the many resources that help awaken transformation and give creative life to a session, only offering soulless beats, drone tones, heavy explanations, and monotonous scripts than induce a passive trance that can't dance with the changes that cook and transform lives.

Cooking Rather Than Looking

In the case examples later presented, each session has the expansion and forms of expression that interactionally arose to fit the unique situation.

Creative therapy emphasizes transformative thermodynamics over psychological dynamics, which is why we spend the least time "looking" (interpreting a situation) and the most time "cooking" (acting to expand and heat the room). Again, in the colder temperatures of a session reside non-emotive talk and detached reflection, the setting most familiar to established schools of practice that dispense the elusive talking cure. Here the least dramatically felt life change is possible and the client is most at risk of being further entrenched in small room discourse and habits. At best a client is invited to swap their impoverished interpretation for a slightly roomier one. At worst, a client goes into the therapy office for help with a problem and comes out with a full-blown mental illness diagnosis. In both cases, clients and practitioners remain chained to the premise that a better label, nametag, interpretation, understanding, narrative excerpt, or story is what changes lives.

Creative therapists waste no time seeking a creative warm-up that provides immediate existential expansion, helping everyone set sail in act two for a whole-body voyage on a vaster sea of change-oriented expression. Here is found the enlivened, creative storm that stands above the humdrum work advocated by the professional norm. To tempest or rest? That is the Shakespearean performance question for a therapist to consider before heading to the second act, but not for too long or else the climatic condition for change shall pass.

In the hottest temperatures all preconceived helping methods are transcended in favor of a healing means that is devoted to the most dramatic form of cooking change. Breaking the allegiance and attachment to any institutionalized treatment modality, the vastest locale flies past professional licensure in favor of censuring all that stands in the way of getting to the big room. Here creative therapists become empty vessels for the creative life force, ready to utilize or ignore whatever resources any therapy or healing orientation might provide, without being unnecessarily influenced or restricted by any. This is the rarified air and the creative flair found in a cooked creative therapy session taking place in the highest heat.

Act Three: Returning the Client to the Everyday

No matter how heated and spacious the room becomes, each creative therapy session ends with a transition to the third and final act. Its corresponding operation is the careful design and effective administration of a unique therapeutic prescription for action designed to carry the room expansion, creative heat, and experienced transformation into the daily life of the client. An assigned creative task or uncommon ritual helps extend, heighten, deepen, and advance what was built, evoked, and warmly felt. Without this altered action, the room of the client's life may too quickly shrink and cool in the return to former daily routines and relational habits, like a deep-sea diver getting the bends. The prescription is the finale that keeps the wheel of change turning in a virtuous direction after the client walks out the door.

A creative therapy prescription recommends action that places one foot inside the former everyday room and another foot inside the big room built in the session. Ideally, the prescription should carry enough tension between both worlds so that it feels impossible for the client to either wholly accept or wholly reject the assigned action as rational, irrational, meaningful, or absurd. In other words, the creative therapist's prescription casts the net of a change-inducing double bind that cannot be easily escaped by former habits that resist change. Inside the doubly bound creative tension and inaccessible comprehension of a prescription is *felt* the *raison d'être* for the kind of action that helps maintain big room experience.

The techniques involved in creating this kind of prescription have been previously discussed in our books, *Improvisational Therapy* (Keeney, 1991) and *Creative Therapeutic Technique* (H. Keeney & B. Keeney, 2013). Like mastering any other performance art, it behooves one to gain a lot of practice in designing prescriptions. Long ago, Brad once invented over 1,000 different interventions for one common presenting problem—weight control (he ran an experimental cybernetic weight control project funded by the National Science Foundation)—doing this as a means of developing his performance chops. Here's an example: "Every time you lose weight donate five dollars to a political organization you agree with. Every time you gain weight in a week, donate five dollars to a political organization you find most disagreeable. If needed, write a letter explaining how you disagree with them." Taking the time to invent various uncommon tasks outside of actual sessions helps a therapist develop the ability to invent them on the spot with a client.

We have not stopped practicing the skill of creating prescriptions. Remember that the prescription is the final big moment of a session and as the saying goes—all is well that ends well. As the skill of making creative prescriptions is acquired, keep in mind that canned and premade interventions quickly lose their nutritional change value. Likewise, practicing their construction in a small room can lead to becoming skilled at making chilly fizzlers rather that heat extenders. The best way to prevent this is with the following strategy: after a session is over, try to take a few extra moments to come up with alternative prescriptions while you are still existentially in the big room. If you imagine one you wished you'd given or think of something to add to the one you gave, then contact the client by text or email. Or send a postcard like we often do that gives the prescription an extra booster shot. For a super surprise, we quite frequently record a mini-musical production that we send to the client, delivering another surprise from the big room.

When practicing the invention of prescriptions make sure that you have first invented a big room that can meaningfully host it, even if you have to make up a session with transitions through the first three acts. Or do it backwards: construct an intervention and then imagine a session that ideally fits it. The performance art of creative therapy calls for investing more time building your technical chops than elaborating pre- and post hoc interpretation.

In the sessions that follow, we advise a grown son to grow half a beard and show the other clean-shaven side of his face to his mother whenever he wants a slice of pie, suggest to a man complaining about depression that he should build a house for a feather lost in his childhood, instruct a grown man to carry around a lightning bolt, and coach a psychosomatic woman to have a romantic relationship with her intestine, among other prescriptions. Each session offers a unique plan of action for the client to do something they never previously imagined doing before. This provides a practical and dramatically noticeable way to keep the room of their daily life large and more available for continuing changes. The very act of assigning and discussing the details of the prescription with the client helps reinforce the big room that was built, charge the task with the creative life force and action-oriented meaning, and graciously punctuate the closing and exit of a session. Assigning a task helps keep the conversation focused until the end, preventing any unintentional dismantling of the new constructed reality through conversational drift. It's okay if the client expresses any mix of feelings about the prescription including excitement, joy, nervous anticipation, curiosity, healthy skepticism, elation, humor, or more. What matters is that the client leaves the session feeling as if they have been given an important, life-changing experiment that is congruent with the room size, temperature, and emotional tone of the session.

One of the common traps is for a therapist to be accidentally tripped or led into another therapist's shrink-wrap. A therapy colleague or associate might want to discuss a session you formally or informally mentioned and inquire whether the client's symptom went away or whether you think any meds are temporarily needed. The second you take such a question too seriously, you fall down a tragic rabbit hole and find yourself amongst the pathologists and pharmacologists rather than the creative performers of change. Such a question is more than a request for information; it is sometimes an ill-intentioned big room deflation or an invitation to join the professional shrinks who reside in a small sanatorium where creativity is immediately tied down and sedated. Better to remember the big room you chose to work in and absurdly respond, "My client's symptom had a jolly good time. It gave me a tip on the next horse race."

The same contest between shrunken rooms and vast rooms can sometimes arise when the client returns for the next session. It's essential to not undo the reality that was built and the change that was set in motion by asking them to evaluate their initial condition like they are at a medical doctor's office. Instead, immediately go to the big room that was built in the previous session. No matter what the client says at the beginning of the session, do what you have to do to move everyone back in the big room ASAP. Then try to make that room even bigger than before, utilizing whatever newly arises to keep the wheel turning in the right direction. Every session is the first session with one difference—the last session gave the gift of an already built big room with a virtuous wheel of change.

We once supervised a session at the University of Louisiana and everyone in the room got extremely stuck—the therapist and the whole family. The week before, the adolescent boy had gotten into serious trouble. One calamity after another took place, sinking the whole family into despair and immobility. The session was spinning in a vicious cycle that was making the room smaller by the moment. We then walked into the room and interrupted, asking the most extremely irrational question we would never imagine asking: "Do you all have a ghost living at your house?" Every family member's mouth opened wide and then the mood quickly changed. The mother excitedly replied, "How did you know? Our house is haunted. All of us see ghosts quite often." The session suddenly sprung to life as the family discussed the living dead that were house residents. We designed a prescription that asked them to say some things to the ghosts on our behalf and to invite them to the next session. No one was prepared for the outcome: Many students, including those who hadn't heard anything about the case, sighted numerous ghosts in the clinic and one student even claimed to have videotaped their activity in a session room.

Being creative therapists, we realized that there are far more sources of resources than the conscious mind can imagine or believe. Go as far outside the box as your unconscious recommends and expect the unexpected. Invite the ancestors and while you're at it, why not invite a squirrel and raccoon. We once had a client who was given a prescription to go into the woods and shout to all the creatures, especially the squirrels and raccoons, "I'm back!" We had previously written two random questions on separate pieces of paper, put them in an empty bottle, and tossed it on the floor in front of him. Then we asked him to tip the bottle over and read the question that falls out first. It asked, "Did you ever have a funeral for a pet bunny rabbit?" That's when he told us that not only had he held a funeral for a pet rabbit, he also had many animal friends in his past. Before he got involved with drugs and in trouble with the law, he regularly found comfort sitting in the woods where squirrels and raccoons would walk right up to him with no fear. He talked to them and even brought some of them home as pets. One raccoon trusted him enough to go to school with him for a visit. This was a highly unusual occurrence, even in rural Louisiana. We discovered that he stopped communicating with animals right at the same time that he got into drugs. The young man followed our advice and went back to the woods and announced he was back and would not leave them again. That action ended up being the first step toward his recovery.

When you make a prescription for your client or yourself, consider inviting anyone to the next session. Invite Rumi, Merlin, Our Lady of Guadalupe, Lily Tomlin, or Bugs Bunny. Do it because you have no idea what might happen. You might dream a dream that changes what you do in the next session, or get a glimpse, hear a faint sound, or feel a tapping that reminds you of what they might do if they were there. Go ahead and be proud to intervene and prescribe as a dedicated member of the imaginary creative therapy tribe, unashamed to walk in the woods where a critter might whisper or write on a tree: "You could if you *would* walk more in the *woods*."

Creative therapists will always need to self-prescribe post-session action for themselves because they, too, are at risk for another fall into small and non-creative existential space. Since most of the modern world is psychologically and medically oriented, opportunities for entry into its inner dark sanctum readily abound. The moment either the client or therapist steps into a mini-container—either during or after a session—subsequent thought, communication, and interactions with others will directly or indirectly begin to turn the wheel of change in an impoverishing direction. It is essential that a creative therapist not shrink the room by reversing the virtuous circle into one that is vicious. This wisdom equally applies to all considerations and discussions following a session. Even talking to colleagues or students afterwards requires congruently remaining in the expanded room that was constructed. Interrupt any post-session reflection, evaluation, or explanation that drifts too far from what transpired in the interaction because it risks dragging a conversant back to an antithetical straitjacket of shrunken psychology, sedated psychiatry, toxic medicine, or chilled ideology. It is not possible to be both a shrink(er) and an expander, sometimes acting like a creative therapist and at other times acting like a psychologist, psychiatrist, social worker, coach, or a member of any profession that lacks or bans room expansion and the increased heat needed to cook change. To even consider stepping into such an antithetical role is itself an indication that the leap to creative therapy has not been made.

One night at the beginning of a clinical supervision for graduate students, to help them dare to be different in their sessions, we gave the instruction to begin all sessions that night with the same opening line. We told them to ask this randomly chosen question: "Do you live with a vision?" After rehearsing how to deliver the line with various tones and rhythms, we went to the first scheduled case. As one student went into the clinical room to meet a mother and son, the rest of the team gathered behind a one-way mirror. Before the trainee could ask the opening question, the mother and son started arguing. It kept escalating and the therapist could not get in a single word. We walked into the room and turned off the light and the room went dark. It also went silent. Then we asked very slowly and inquisitively, "Do you live with a vision?" After more silence, the son calmly replied, "Please turn on the light so I can show you my answer." After the light was on he stood and opened his shirt to reveal a tattoo that stretched across his chest. It was a single word: "vision." The rest of the session involved less divisive fission and instead explored the creation of a more uniting vision for the home. The intervention that ended the hour involved making more visible what had been invisible—vision. The mother and son were asked to put on darkly painted sunglasses and close their eyes whenever they needed to remember that they are alive to serve a future vision rather than trigger nuclear family fission. We recommended that the trainees also make themselves the same kind of therapy spectacles, so they'd remember that a session can become clearer when they sit in the dark and welcome a visionary surprise.

Creative therapy sessions are filled with assignments that involve strings, bottles, twigs, leaves, magical drawings, odd objects, collected buttons, scrapbook items, watches that stopped at a certain time, strangely written words, re-captioned family photographs, colored powders, and even uncommon liquid solutions. For instance, we advised a Russian homeopathic doctor to make some marmalade that included the addition of one drop of her own tears that were to be gathered as she longed for her grandmother, someone she enjoyed making marmalade with as a child. This allowed her to put her family sorrow to good medicinal use. You can do the same, whether the medicinal drop is collected from tears of sadness or laughter, depending on the need and jam at home. Not only place a drop of an emotional outcome into a jar, drop yourself in the sea to help wash off whatever debris interferes with smelling the fragrances and tasting the tastes of life. Hold up a glass of air, collected in a happy moment, and say, "Here's to life." Go ahead and have a drink of love, the ultimate potion every healer serves when any other medicine won't go down.

Write this pledge on the back of your driver's license if it helps remind you of all that you can do rather than only view in a session: "I solemnly and absurdly swear to not shrink, stink, or chill the therapy room with psycho-medico babble that goes nowhere instead of tumbling along the open change trail like the cybernetically enhanced tumbleweed I was born to be." Or keep it simple: "Three-Operation Agent of Change." Why not believe that you deserve a better license and diploma than the one that has nothing to do with creative change? Add a "Ch.D." to your name when you think you've earned your doctorate of changeology. Milton Erickson would and did in our fantasy reality, so you can feel free to do the same.

If needed, wear a new ring on a formerly unbetrothed finger that now is your reminder to steadfastly travel around the circle of change rather than risk getting lost and imprisoned inside another theoretical model. When you notice yourself or others going into Pandora's box of hermeneutics, call upon Hermes, the Greek trickster god who was also the patron protector of journeys. Do this while allowing a finger to touch and circle the ring, demonstrating that you are in a committed relationship with the creative life force and its ecstatic pulse.

Big room change realigns therapeutic action with the creative force that can transform any wear or tear while warming the heart. Whenever pain is transfigured into joy, the creative therapist and client learn more about the gardener's mystery of life—wherever there is a thorn, a beautiful rose waits nearby. And where there is a rose there is a whole garden blossoming, made possible by sunshine as well as rain. Lasting fulfillment is not found in the absence of suffering, the avoidance of pain, or the illusory pursuit of perfection, but in rebuilding one's relationship to vastness and re-directing the wheel of change so it can turn in a virtuous direction, finding the way back to the big room for another round of being hooked and cooked by change.

Creative therapy sessions provide clients with the opportunity to fulfill their destiny as a recipient, ambassador, and teacher of change. We are grateful to all our clients who have helped deliver to the world a new kind of true fairy tale that celebrates how sunshine comes through no matter how cloudy conditions may initially appear. As both creative therapists and their clients become accustomed to building big rooms, getting experientially cooked by change, and conducting uncommon experiments with life, they will become more naturally attuned to setting this process in motion whenever they find themselves viciously stuck in a creatively lifeless space. Through ongoing entry and re-entry into the big room, more of life is illumined, enlightening how even amidst the mayhem, everyone's life can joyfully blossom and come to fruition.

Your prescription can also be more literal to assure that your metaphors don't pull you away from expanding the space. Go ahead and make a sign that spells out: "The Big Room" and then hang it up in your therapy room. Make one for your kitchen, too, and any other room needing expansion and creative warmth. Do it to remember where you need to be and that every medicine produced and taken needs to help get you there.

Becoming a Creative Therapist

Like a traditional healer of old, becoming a creative therapist requires ongoing practice, experimentation, and skill development, but it also requires an initiatory experience that establishes a more immediately felt relationship with a big room. Although life has already been tenderizing and seasoning everyone since birth, there is another kind of creative transformation available that is only made possible through being cooked at a higher temperature. This is when we say that a therapist is rewired and made a healer, something we have addressed elsewhere (H. Keeney & B. Keeney, 2012a). Until that time comes, however, a practitioner can prepare by acting without the use of any former crutch or training wheel. Become theoretically free, empty of narrative, cleared of interpretation, and absent of the filter of any dominating view. Be less mindful of mind and fuller of the kind of heartfelt emotion that reaches for the creative life force. Anything less cannot embody the higher-order changing of change.

Creative therapy's performed creative elation is a healing negation of any former exaltation of an abstract scheme detached from the experiential stream. At the same time, it brings an experienced confirmation and expressed affirmation of a big room's wholeness, as the ineffable is infused into all who enter its boundless space. Here we find that the missing piece of a client's life and the missing piece of a therapist's practice are not pieces at all. What's gone missing is an experience of the forever changing, always evolving, and constantly revolving whole.

Emphasizing creative action over theoretical interpretation, hunting for the ecstatic pulse of the creative life force, expanding the room, turning up its temperature, getting cooked by change, and being more experimental in the everyday comprise more than a new way of doing therapy. This is a whole new way of living. The creative therapist seeks to become more like an electrical lightning rod that helps bring down the current of change. This conductance, both electrical and theatrical, does not merely add another healing method to the familiar, eclectic medicine cabinet. It offers a different room in which to work and live. Unless you've been cooked by change in a big room, you haven't yet met what is possible beyond common talk and its mundane walk. Past the heard and the seen are the unheard and the unseen unknown that can only be felt until its sound and scene make real a new kind of performed dream.

Here's some action to help get your creative juices circulating. After a day of seeing clients, write down the most creative metaphor for each client you saw. We actually name our clients this way—we have clients named Pigeon Lady, Lightning King, Apple Cake Baker, Bee Man, Mr. America, Seiki Girl, Ghost Family, Feather Man, The Light Man, The Green Light, The Woman Who Married Jerusalem, Magmore, and so on. These names are both playful and honorific because they reflect the primary "change metaphors" that arose in their sessions. Do the same for the clients you worked with this day. Now fold up the list and place it in an empty ice tray. Fill it with water and place it in the freezer. The following week on the day these clients are scheduled to return, take the ice tray out when you get up in the morning. Set it near a window where sunshine can pour over it throughout the day. When you go to your sessions, and especially when you are conducting them, remember that the ice is melting, and your metaphors are undergoing a thaw. You, too, can step out of the therapy freezer and have yourself a good creative melt. Why not keep a glass of ice in the room where you see clients? Rather than wonder what you need to know about a client, take action and watch the ice melt. Ask the client to join you because a therapist and client experiencing a melt together are more likely to make the session alive rather than talk a room to death.

Creative therapy courageously warns against following any helping profession that offers little more than a license to spiritually chill, more likely making ill the room within which practitioners and clients meet. It takes many crossings into the big room to make a therapist more prepared to creatively turn and burn whatever needs to change. The conductance of change and its transforming ability to alter whatever falters cannot surface unless a therapist is willing to learn how to expand the surrounding space, tap into the ecstatic pulse, and welcome the change that cooks.

Notes

1 Whitaker repeatedly stated that there is no such thing as an individual; the term only indicates a family fragment. Cited in Gary Connell, Tammy Mitten, and William M. Bumberry, *Reshaping Family Relationships: The Symbolic Therapy of Carl Whitaker*, Philadelphia, PA: Bruner/Mazel, 1998, p. 27.

2 For more on cybernetics and its unique recursive form of circularity that we are here calling a "wheel of change" see *Aesthetics of Change* (1983) and *Circular Therapeutics: Giving Therapy a Healing Heart* (2012a).

PART II
Creative Therapy Case Studies

We regard every session as an opportunity to create a unique and valuable experience for all involved. Rather than be limited by the idea that creative therapy should only try to "fix," "cure," or "solve," we prefer regarding each session as the birthplace of a profound process of change that will circulate throughout the room and even beyond its walls. We act as if a client is "chosen" by their relational ecosystem or the universe at large to deliver an important communication, a fascinating teaching, and a unique prescription of action to the world. Accordingly, we convey the curiosity of co-exploration and the anticipation of an exciting shared journey instead of posturing the elevated and removed position of observation, diagnosis, or explanation. The issue, challenge, problem, symptom, or suffering that rallied someone to seek our help is tacitly regarded as a messenger, a representative, a scout, or an ally of change. We respect and appreciate its role in the scheme of it all while also trying to communicate that it has accomplished its important job of gathering people for a session, which is already a sign that the clients are ready to move on with their lives. As the following sessions demonstrate, the creative therapist aims to make room for resourceful changes to spontaneously unfold and proliferate, the creative dynamic that changes lives. This is something that benefits others who witness or participate in what transpires. At the end of each of the following transcribed sessions we discuss the newborn teaching that can be applied to you and your own creative therapeutic work.

Often confused, struggling, and clinging to old habits of thought and deed, clients come to sessions with a history of consciously or unconsciously ignoring or pushing back whatever gift and teaching their situation is attempting to hatch. Unfortunately, traditionally schooled therapists assume clients are in a battle with an enemy or pathogenic agent rather than going through a process of change that began with the rise of a discomforting experience. Hence their pursuit of medical-like evaluation, psychological explanation, psychiatric classification, and the reification and externalization of a problem metaphor in order to justify extracting or going to war with challenging experience. The creative therapist avoids such connotation in order to respectfully meet and greet the issue as a systemic communication in need of a healthier interaction that aims to evolve rather than solve the situation. When the messenger (i.e. the problem) is blocked or fought, its call for change is amplified with greater urgency. Though too often mistaken for a clinical emergency, it is actually another opportunity for growth. Instead of responding with immediate banishment or rage, a symptom or problem needs a bigger stage that allows it to express what's benevolent and resourceful. A therapist engaging in warfare with any part of a client's experience deserves a one-way ticket to the Middle Ages where inquisitions and exorcisms belong (see H. Keeney & B. Keeney, 2012b).

A vicious cycle ensues when the messenger and its unconscious means of communication are disrespected and attacked rather than welcomed for the gifts they are designed to bring forth. Suffering is often more attributable to resisting reception of what the more encompassing circle of life brings to the front door, even if it arrives as shocking, confusing, disappointing, tragic, or painful. The resourceful contributions of an ordeal only emerge when the room becomes big enough for change to ignite and cook. A creative therapist needs a creative emergence-room, not a clinical emergency room. Each session then provides a unique opportunity for the midwifery of transformation. Here creative change is inseparable from the vibrant force of creation that breaks new ground and sprouts the unexpected. We celebrate the amazing teaching and remarkable gifts every session brings to us and we are grateful to be able to share them with others.

4

HALF A BEARD WITH A SLICE OF SOUR CHERRY PIE

This session was conducted in front of an audience in Budapest, Hungary with a 34-year-old man named Gábor, and his mother, Eszter. When they arrived and were seated, Brad immediately went to the piano and began to play, melodically speaking to Eszter and Gábor while accompanied by improvised music. Both mother and son were visibly touched and delighted by this surprise, and it moved the audience to tears. The room was immediately wrapped in tender heartfelt sounds, carrying us swiftly to a vaster performance ground.

BRAD: This is just a little music for you, as my way of saying, "Hello."

GÁBOR: [Smiling and nodding shyly] Thank you.

HILLARY: It is also our way of saying, "Thank you for coming," because we see that you are both alive. Whatever has happened to you, we see that you're alive.
[Son and mother both nod and smile]

GÁBOR: Yes, yes.
[Brad now sings his words. The music is like a sweet lullaby]

BRAD: Isn't it something,
that you're alive?
All these years,
you're still together.
All the things that have happened to you,
you still can smile.
You still have joy in your hearts.
Life is full of so many challenges.

	Not everybody gets through, but you are here. Which tells us you are strong, very, very strong.
GÁBOR:	[Nodding and smiling] Yes, yes.
BRAD:	We celebrate you. We say, "Thank you." I wish I could write you a song, about a mother and a son, a mother who gave birth to the moon. And he said, when he grew up, "I'm not the moon, I'm your sun."
GÁBOR:	[Mother and son are both smiling] Yes.
BRAD:	You are the light, of your mother's life. She gave birth to light. Mother's light, and mother's sun. [Brad brings the melody to a close. The room is filled with even more tenderness and emotion. Brad sits down next to Hillary]
GÁBOR:	[Smiling] Thank you.
ESZTER:	[Smiling, with tears in her eyes] Thank you.
HILLARY:	Welcome. Please share what you would like.
ESZTER:	He is sick.
BRAD:	And you are taking care of him?
ESZTER:	Yes, I take care of him one hundred percent.
BRAD:	So, you are his doctor, his nurse, and his mother?
ESZTER:	I'm the mother, I am the provider, and I am his caretaker.
HILLARY:	So, what is healthy about your son? I ask because I see that he has a healthy smile.
ESZTER:	I don't know. [Eszter looks at her son as if to invite him to respond]
GÁBOR:	I don't know. Maybe my body, but I don't know.
BRAD:	[Speaking to Eszter] But you have seen his healthy smile, yes?
ESZTER:	Yes.
BRAD:	Because some mothers have a son, especially at his age, who have an unhealthy smile. But he has a healthy smile.
ESZTER:	It's rare that he smiles. He does not smile often.
BRAD:	[Speaking to Gábor] Ah, so this smile is a rare thing for you to share. [Gábor shrugs his shoulders. He is rocking back and forth slightly in his chair]

ESZTER: He is depressed and sad a lot. I cheer him up. That's what I do; I try to cheer him up. I always try to say and do happy things. I put color in his life.

BRAD: Can I say something? [Brad turns to Gábor] I'm going to give you a different diagnosis. From what I have seen already, you are a son who hides his smile. You keep it hidden.

GÁBOR: [Nodding] Yes, yes.

HILLARY: There are probably times when you want to smile, but you don't.

GÁBOR: Yes.

BRAD: It takes a lot of work to be someone who really knows how to give a great smile. Don't hold it back. It's as if you play hide and seek with your smile. You hide it and your mother has to find out where you hid it. Your mother has to try many ways to find it, such as baking you a special pie.

ESZTER: [Upon hearing this Eszter straightens up in her chair and nods emphatically] Yes, I do bake him pie. Every day I bake him a sour cherry pie. Every day.

[Mother and son look at each other and laugh. The audience also laughs]

BRAD: So, both of you play hide and seek.

ESZTER: He is sad very often. He is always tired, and he lies down a lot.

BRAD: Yes, but from now on—at least for the next few minutes—I invite you to accept my professional diagnosis that the two of you are playing hide and seek. He hides his smile and you seek it. This way he gets a lot of pie.

[Brad smiles, everyone laughs]

HILLARY: Yes. This is the way that very, very big love is expressed.

ESZTER: He has a dog that is 15 years old. He is always petting the dog and it cheers him up. He loves the dog a lot. If he wants to be in a good mood, he goes to the dog and pets it and hugs it.

BRAD: Of course; because he is normal.

GÁBOR: [Nodding] Normal.

BRAD: If your son pets the dog and cried, then he would be sick. But he pets the dog and feels happy, this tells me that you are playing hide and seek. I want to say something right now because I see how open both of you are. I would usually wait for a long time to say this, but instead I'm going to say it right now. [Brad turns to Gábor] You're hiding a lot of things from your mom. You are even hiding your age. How old are you?

GÁBOR: Thirty-four.

BRAD: [Brad holds his hand up to the side of his face as if to prevent Eszter from hearing, then whispers] Shhhhh. She might hear. It's a secret.

[Eszter and the audience chuckle]

GÁBOR: [Smiling] Yes.

BRAD: Sometimes she thinks you are twelve.

GÁBOR: [Nodding and speaking emphatically] Yes, yes.

ESZTER: What's more, I often tell him he behaves like a five-year-old kindergartener.

BRAD: [To Gábor] Wow, you hide very well. Congratulations!

ESZTER: I don't want to embarrass him by saying this, but sometimes he'll say to me, "I'm going to use the bathroom" or "I'm going to go wash my hands," but I tell him, "You don't have to tell me that; you are an adult."

BRAD: But that's how he hides. [To Gábor] That's how you hide your age.

GÁBOR: Yes. Sorry, I'm a little nervous and a little anxious right now [Gábor is rocking back and forth in his chair and shaking his hands]

HILLARY: That's fine because that's also a part of hiding. It's a good way to hide, because it would be very shocking to your mother if, for example, you grew a long beard.

GÁBOR: [Smiles and nods] Yes.

HILLARY: She would see that and say, "Whoa! A five-year-old with a beard!" [Audience laughs] If you did that you would make her feel very crazy.

GÁBOR: [Smiling] Yes.

BRAD: Maybe you should grow half a beard. Then you could go into the kitchen and show your mother the side of your face with no beard, and say, "I'm sad, I want pie." Then, when you go to the table to eat the pie you could show her the side with the beard and say [Brad speaks in a low, manly voice], "I want all of the pie. I'm a man." [Eszter and Gábor chuckle] That would be very interesting, yes? I think I know what you need in order to make your life more interesting. I don't think you're sad. I think you get bored.

GÁBOR: [Nodding] Yes, yes.

BRAD: You get so bored that it makes you sad. You feel sad, but you're really bored.

ESZTER: He has depression.

HILLARY: Nope, not depression. It's hide and seek. [Speaking now to Gábor] You are bored, which sometimes make you sad, so you play hide and seek. I want to make your game more interesting. Do you ever go out by yourself, or does your mother always take you out?

GÁBOR: Once a week I go out on Sundays and meet a friend who I was in the psychiatric hospital with. Otherwise, I am always at home.

BRAD: What I'm going to say will sound totally crazy, but I'm going to say it anyway because I see enough life in you. I see your smile and I see how smart you are in order to get all that pie. [Mother, son, and audience laugh] I want to ask you to make history. I don't want to disturb what you have going on here; I just want you to go all the way and make history. I want you to go to a costume shop and buy a beard. Buy a beard—the kind that you can wear—and cut half of it off.

GÁBOR: Okay, yes.

BRAD: Really. And then, when you're with your mother—

GÁBOR: Or maybe I could grow one.

HILLARY: Perfect. Even better. But start with the fake one, and then let your face catch up.

GÁBOR: Would I look better with a beard do you think?

HILLARY: That question is for later. We'll ask that question later. For now, you need half a beard. Because if you get a whole beard, you'll lose the pie. Right now, you are addicted to pie. [Brad smiles]

GÁBOR: [Nodding enthusiastically and smiling] Yes, yes.

BRAD: Yes, therefore we don't want the pie to go away too fast. First, your mother needs to see you with only half a beard. She still needs to see some of your clean-shaven face. [Brad studies Gábor's face] I can see that you give yourself a very clean shave. Even this late in the day I see that you maintain a very clean shave.

GÁBOR: Yes, I do. But today I made a slight mistake right here. [Gábor points to a place on his cheek where he missed a spot, but it is barely visible]

BRAD: [Studying Gábor's face] Ah yes, I see. So, you have already begun the experiment. That tells me that this side of your face should be the baby face, and this side should have the beard. [Brad points to the side where Gábor said he missed a spot] Let's try it right now. [Brad turns Gábor's head to one side, so that only one side of his face is shown to his mother]. Right now, she only sees the baby face. Now, turn the other way. [Gábor turns his head and shows his mother the other side] On this side, he has a beard. [Brad speaks to Eszter] This is going to shock you, Mother, because he will have to decide which side he will hide—the side with the beard, or the side without. I think it would be best to do this experiment when the sun goes down—right at the time when the day is ending, and the night is beginning—because that is the time of day when things change. That's when you, Gábor, should be fully dressed with half a beard, and turn your head from side to side. You can experiment with various angles and different sides. [Brad makes the action of showing different sides of his face in relationship to Gábor.] You can even change where you sit in relationship to your mother. And while you are conducting this experiment, go ahead and grow your real beard.

GÁBOR: Yes, okay.

BRAD: Can I recruit you to be the first man in the history of the world to do this?

GÁBOR: [Smiling and nodding] Yes.

HILLARY: Wonderful! We have an historic experiment! You will be the first man to have half a beard and hide both of your ages from your mother. Your mother is to pretend she never heard any of this. [The audience laughs and Eszter smiles. Brad now whispers to Gábor]

BRAD: When she sees this side of your face [pointing to the clean-shaven side] she'll want to bake the pies. But when she sees this side of your face [pointing to the side with the beard] she might say, "I'm tired, why don't you go get *me* a pie!" [Brad gasps as if in shock. His eyes grow wide and his voice becomes a quiet, yet intense whisper] Whoa! It will get very wild in your house! You will get to be all things. You might even practice having half a smile [Brad tries to make half a smile, and everyone erupts in laughter. Gábor tries it also and the audience claps] So how soon can you get the beard? Do you know where there is a costume shop in Budapest?

GÁBOR: No.

HILLARY: You'll have to look on the internet.

GÁBOR: Yes, I can do that.

BRAD: You should do it fast! [Brad claps his hands together once, loudly]

GÁBOR: Can I walk on the street with it?

BRAD: That's up to you. I don't know.

ESZTER: He is not allowed to contact women in public. For example, yesterday he was on the subway, and when he came home he was upset because a woman on the subway was looking at him. It made him very upset and nervous. I said to him, "It was probably because she liked you, because you are at the age when that can happen."

HILLARY: Yes, because he is playing hide and seek again.

GÁBOR: I think it doesn't make sense to get to know someone or make a relationship while I am sick.

BRAD: When you play hide and seek like that, it means there is no beard. You're right—now is not the time to talk about your life while you're growing the beard. That's for later. I'm not sure how long your beard will have to grow. Maybe you'll have to have a beard that grows all the way to the ground before we can talk about such things. [Gábor and audience laugh] But that's a long way away. It's nothing to worry about now. Just focus on this experiment. I think it has to happen soon—perhaps Monday or Tuesday. Get your costume beard, cut it in half, and start your experiment. [Turning to mother] And don't forget, he still wants the pies. So, if you see half a beard, don't think that this means he doesn't want the pie. He still wants the pie.

ESZTER: It is so interesting that you are talking to him about a beard. A month ago, he asked me, "What would you think if I grew a beard? How do you think it would look? I'm thinking of growing one." I was totally against it. [Mother laughs, and so does the audience]

HILLARY: He is so ahead of all of us. Don't worry; he's only going to have half a beard for now. He will keep one side of his face the same, so he can continue to have the pie.

ESZTER: And what are people going to say if he steps out into the street like that, with half a beard?

BRAD: This is about making history! He will decide when it's time to go into the street. [Gábor shows excitement and is nodding.] People might think he is a famous actor rehearsing for a part. There are all kinds of creative things people might think. People might wonder what kind of special mother this man has, because she gave him the courage to walk around in the world any way he wants. But you, Gábor, will decide when the time is right for that. We are going to call you on Monday or Tuesday to make sure that this experiment is moving forward, and that you are on your way to getting the beard. It's very important.

GÁBOR: What if I can't find one? Then can I grow one?

HILLARY: First, you should find one. It's out there somewhere. While you are wearing half the costume beard, you can grow your real one at the same time. I don't want you to wait. Let me put it this way: You need to wear half the beard as a dress rehearsal for when you have a whole beard. Okay?

GÁBOR: Okay.

BRAD: When we hear that you have done this, that this is happening, and that history is being made, I'm going to record a song for you.

GÁBOR: [Smiles] Thank you.

BRAD: Yes, a song about hide and seek and special pies and growing a beard.

GÁBOR: Okay, thank you.

HILLARY: Wonderful! It's time for you to begin the experiment.
[Brad nods and he and Hillary stand. After Brad embraces Eszter, she takes hold of Brad's hand and asks him a question]

ESZTER: But can I still bake the pies?

BRAD AND HILLARY: [In unison] Yes! Of course! Absolutely!
[The audience laughs with delight. They clap as Gábor and Eszter exit, waving to everyone as they walk by]

This session brought the surprise of sour cherry pie and half a beard, teaching us that no one ever fully grows up because we are always some mother's child—a boy or girl to the one who brought us across the birth canal. This is true even if a mother is no longer physically alive or was never known. The umbilical bond with a mother is a biological truth that lasts forever, and this means that it is good to honor its contribution to the continuance of life. During holidays or home visits, it is practically wise to respectfully show the child-side of the face. Mothers, or those temporarily stepping into the role, are then able to serve pie and provide the assurance that children always need to hear. At the same time this gives mothers what they need to receive from their offspring.

The other side of everyone's face is that of an adult. There a beard or lipstick may decorate this difference. There is a time, place, and face for remaining a child and another time, place, and face for being an adult. When the face of a child or adult appears at the cost of erasing the other side, lives become unbalanced and only half-true. This is true for all relational matters at home, work, and play. Being able to step into the performance role of a child and an adult, shifting from one to the other as the occasion calls for it, is the sign of a more wholesome life. As Carl Whitaker recommended, even the role of scapegoat must be rotated in a family to assure the health of the whole system (as cited in cited in Neill & Kniskern, 1982, p. 275).

The creative therapist also draws upon these shifting faces and masks in a session. Go ahead and serve the client a piece of pie but know that you must also recognize when it is time for a different face and role. Creative therapists must be able to perform mothering and fathering as well as all the other familial roles and more. They must also be able to literally and metaphorically go home and enjoy its desserts like a child. Utilize the wisdom Rudyard Kipling expressed: "God could not be everywhere, and therefore he made mothers." Honor all mothers by both remaining a dependable child and enacting their success—showing that you were raised to also be successfully independent. Similarly, if you were therapeutically reared and steered by a model, someday you and your clients will benefit when you leave home with more faces of change.

What is more important than an awareness of the benefits of accessing child-like and adult-like resources, is taking the *action* that makes this adage a live performance rather than a homespun reflection. We therefore ask you to choose one time a week when you will have a special desert, something delicious that you might have requested when you were a child. Perhaps it's a slice of pie. Think what would have truly pleased you when you were very young. Arrange to have this dessert—make it, request it, or order it at a bakery or café. Then sit down to enjoy this delicacy, remembering all the delight that such a treat formerly brought. Be childlike as the sweetness pleases your taste and memory. However, do not eat more than one-half of this dessert for you have another side of you that is an adult. This side must say, "That is enough time for being a child." Now is the moment for a cup of coffee, tea, mineral water, or whatever the adult nature of you selects. Drink half the cup or glass, being grateful that you are able to choose and enact when to be a child and when to be an adult. This, after all, is one of the secrets of having a more creatively wholesome therapy life.

5

A TRUE FAIRY TALE

This session was conducted privately with Lena and her daughter Rebecca, age fifteen, in New Orleans, Louisiana. The clients flew in from out of state saying that they had an emergency situation that couldn't wait any longer for help. They arrived expressing an urgent need to begin with their story, as if it had never been told to anyone before.

LENA: About ten months ago, I divorced Rebecca's father and moved out of our family home in North Carolina. I took a job in Massachusetts, leaving Rebecca and her older brother at home with their father. Four months ago, Rebecca came to visit me in Massachusetts and this is when I discovered that she had been cutting herself. Rebecca's grades have also been slipping, which is a change for her because she has always been a good student. I became concerned that she is now smoking too much marijuana, skipping school, and not getting enough supervision at home, so I moved back to North Carolina. It's now a bit awkward because we are all living together again, and I'm sleeping on the couch. I still intend to move out at some point. Rebecca and I are arguing a lot and things at home are very tense.

HILLARY: What about you, Rebecca?

REBECCA: When my mom left I was left to take care of everything at home. My brother is eighteen, has a car, and lives his own life. He has freedom. My dad has been drinking a lot and takes antidepressants. I had to take care of him when she left.

LENA: Rebecca has had to grow up very fast since all this happened. I worry about her getting involved with the wrong crowd.

She has become too isolated and spends too much time alone in her room. Her grades are slipping.

REBECCA: That's because you won't let me leave the house. You're always nagging and saying I need supervision, asking me where I'm going. She is on my back all the time. I don't understand her logic or thinking behind it—she worries that I'm too isolated, but then she doesn't want me out with friends.

LENA: I don't trust that you won't skip school and smoke pot. Her new social group is the kids that don't do well in school.

REBECCA: They're the stoners, I admit. But Mom I'm actually worried about *you* being too isolated. [Rebecca and Lena both laugh] My mother is really uptight and weird—my brother and I used to try to give her lessons on how to be more cool [Lena and Rebecca both laugh]

HILLARY: Lena, tell us something extraordinary about Rebecca.

LENA: She is a wonderful poet and short story writer.

HILLARY: Really, wow! [Rebecca looks at her mother and smiles]

LENA: Also, I was in labor with Rebecca for almost two days and the doctors were concerned that I would not survive her birth. Giving birth to her was an extraordinary ordeal. The other thing interesting about Rebecca is that when she was two years old my husband had to go to China for work and we went with him. It was crazy because wherever we went, all of the locals kept lining up to hold her and have their pictures taken with her. [Lena and Rebecca laugh]

HILLARY: Here she is now, already a poet and writer, trying to figure out how to transition or birth herself from childhood to young adulthood. Of course, this will be an extraordinary process, because we are talking about Rebecca. [Turning to Rebecca] Given the facts of your life, from your extraordinary birth to the way you were mysteriously celebrated as a child in China, we guess there are many interesting and extraordinary things about you. Perhaps there is some interesting reason that you have chosen to hook up with this new social group. Maybe you're conducting an experiment.

LENA: She is very interested in how the brain works—

REBECCA: [Interrupting] That's right, and how thinking works and memory is stored and why people do the things they do.

LENA: There is something to what you just said—it's almost like her new group of friends provides a little experiment for her to study "the dark side" and to have an experience of being submerged in that world.

BRAD: Rebecca, perhaps you are like an undercover experimental behavioral researcher.

REBECCA: [Smiles and chuckles] Yes, exactly.

LENA: That's part of what makes me nervous. When I was a teenager, exploring my "edge" meant going on wilderness experiences. My mother used to worry about me because I would ask to go on these expeditions in the freezing north where it would be 60 degrees below zero and we'd be sleeping outside and testing the water samples under the ice for oxygen levels because this was in the early days of researching acid rain.

HILLARY: Wow, you really are weird! [Rebecca, Lena, and Brad laugh]

LENA: That was my big excitement as a teenager. My mom supported that, even though I'm sure she was a bit scared. It was dangerous, but I loved it. I had the moral compass of my spiritual background and my relationship with nature. Now it's a struggle for me to see Rebecca struggling in this milieu without a compass. I'm sure she has one, but I can't see it from the outside. I mean that she's a devout atheist.

REBECCA: I am not a devout atheist. I just don't have a strong belief in anything.

LENA: It just makes me nervous. Rebecca has a high tolerance for danger. Her tolerance for danger is much higher than mine.

HILLARY: It sounds like both of you are scientists. Maybe Rebecca is your experiment, and Lena, perhaps you are Rebecca's experiment. You are each experimentally studying the other. [Rebecca and Lena laugh] I say this because I think you are both very curious about each other. Earlier, Rebecca essentially expressed an interest in how you, Mom, cognitively track her situation. She wants to know how you put all this together in your mind.

REBECCA: That's right. With my dad, I always feel very clear about the logic behind his thinking. I consider myself a very logical person. But Mom, I find it difficult to listen to you sometimes, because you just say, "Do this, do that," and I want to know the logic behind it. You just say, "Because."

BRAD: You want to see more of the underlying cognitive, logical structure behind it.

REBECCA: Yes, I want to know why.

LENA: I come at things more intuitively. Rebecca wanted to know why we were coming all the way to New Orleans, for example, to see you both when we could have gone to a therapist in our city.

BRAD: Good question. Perhaps you came here so you can see the crazy life in New Orleans. It's Mardi Gras time.

REBECCA: Now I have a photo of my mom catching Mardi Gras beads at last night's parade. [Lena laughs]

HILLARY: This is a very irrational city, especially during Mardi Gras.

BRAD: This is good for both of you. You both seem so rational. You both speak so scientifically, and what upsets you is when things are not laid out rationally. Probably the best thing for you right now is to be here in the height of Mardi Gras irrationality. Right now, this is the most irrational place on earth.

[Hillary gets up and puts on a Mardi Gras mask as Brad goes to the keyboard and plays some jazz in a New Orleans manner]

REBECCA: See Mom? The best thing for us to do is to just go crazy.

BRAD [SINGING]: That's a great idea, because the blues mixed with some Mardi Gras beads and syncopation makes good mojo. The crazier your jazz is here, the better the medicine.

REBECCA: I keep telling her that, to just be sporadic. I urge her to do stuff she's never done before just because she can.

HILLARY: What would be an example of that? If your mom really went crazy in a good way and found liberation tonight, what would she do?

[Hillary has moved to a pair of drums and now plays a drum roll before Rebecca answers]

REBECCA: She would have to do something crazy that she's never done before, like shave her legs or part her hair normally, or go out to a bar, and not eat dinner at six, but eat dinner at eight o'clock just because she can! [Rebecca and Lena erupt in laughter.]

BRAD: Awesome! [Hillary makes a cymbal crash!] Mom, you have quite a coach!

REBECCA: But she'd never do it.

HILLARY: Why not? I think it's a good experiment for you to see whether or not you are able to convince her to do something she doesn't normally do. You have to convince her that it's an interesting experiment. She'd do it for science. Or she'd do it for spirituality, since she believes in all that stuff.

[Brad plays a clock sound on the synthesizer: tick tock tick tock …]

REBECCA: We'll document it. [Rebecca turns to her mother] Mom, get in touch with your inner spirit by experimenting with the other side, because there is no happiness without sadness, you have to mix the two!

HILLARY: [Addressing Lena] Wow! [Cymbal crash!] She sounds like a crazy wisdom teacher. Rebecca, I thought you'd suggest something far more extreme for your mother to do.

REBECCA: Nah, I'd never make her do something too crazy. Little steps. Little steps are best. [Rebecca and Lena giggle]

HILLARY: Well there's a compass. That's quite a wisdom compass.

REBECCA: When my mom was little, she got straight As and was a "good" teenager. For me to be me, I need to experiment with myself. I need to have more of that rebel–bad–other side of society stuff. While other people tend to look down on it, I feel that it's something I need. That's why my dad and I get along right now, because he doesn't nag at me as much. He just tells me to make sure I don't get arrested. Sometimes people do get arrested for the kinds of things my friends do, but I still feel I need to do those things in order to be like a rebel child.

HILLARY: Two things come to my mind right now. The first is, when we asked you, Rebecca, for an example of what it would mean for your mother to go wild, you suggested some of the tamest things anyone could think of. Lena, you're worried about your daughter going wild, but the wildest things she can recommend for you are shaving your legs, changing the part of your hair, and going to a bar? [Lena and Rebecca laugh]

HILLARY: Second, Rebecca has got quite a compass. Furthermore, it sounds as if all of this is kind of like a science project.

BRAD: [Speaking to Rebecca] All of this has something to do with helping you survive being bored to death. It actually sounds like you are doing something that is more than a science. [Brad switches to a melodic and melodramatic vocal tone] It sounds spiritual, magical, metaphysical, experimental, or autobiographical.

REBECCA: Yep, like a self-quest kind of thing.

BRAD: Since your mom is also a scientist, maybe you have been going about it wrong. Maybe you should recruit your mom to investigate all of this with you. You could decide to do it together. I don't know what that means, but let's just fantasize about that for fun right now.

HILLARY: Let's make something up. What if your mom got over whatever it is that she's doing that's annoying you. Let's just assume for now that we all know what that is, even though for both of you it's different. Rebecca, for you it's nagging and Mom, for you it's just trying to be a good parent. What if instead of all that, Mom just said, "Rebecca, let's research this together." It would be like taking an expedition to the Arctic and coming back with data. Maybe your mom could sometimes go undercover, and sometimes you would do the same. You could disguise your Mom in an undercover scene, perhaps as a street person or some random person hanging out at the corner. The two of you could approach this as if it were an anthropology project where you study other people.

BRAD: Of course both of you would have to monitor the risks involved in your research, like they do in all scientific explorations. For example, you know that if you stay out too late in one area it might get dangerous, or if you do certain things you could get arrested. You have to take those things into consideration as you conduct your research. If you don't cover all the bases, you can get into all sorts of trouble or get arrested, and then it's no longer research, it's just a mess.

REBECCA: Right.

HILLARY: I'd also like to point out that I've never heard a teenager talk so rationally and scientifically about being a rebel.

REBECCA: [Laughing] I get that a lot.

BRAD: Yes, it's like she's developing her own research course, because school is too boring. The other subject of this exploration, as much as anything else, is irrationality. That's perhaps a better word for describing the other side. Because "dark" doesn't really describe anything you can focus on. It leaves you in the dark. Isn't it really irrationality that you're interested in? You are so accustomed to being comfortable with rationality, that what you understand the least is irrationality. You are really engaged in innovative scholarship about the irrational.

REBECCA: Right. Yes. That would be a good title for a book. [Lena and Rebecca laugh.]

HILLARY: There are so many things that have happened in your life over the past year that have been irrational. Things have been tossed about in such a way to pave the way for you to be able to conduct this experiment.

BRAD: This may also have something to do with the destiny that brought the two of you here to New Orleans during Mardi Gras, the capital and holiday of irrationality. When you look back at all the experiments you've had with yourself in your room and outside of it, you can see it as fascinating scholarship. Now that you see more about what this really is, it gives you a different way to think about it, talk about it, and relate to it. Let us remember how bright and creative you really are, and how you came into the world—which was exceptional.

HILLARY: Not to mention the way the people in China saw something special about you.

BRAD: Since there are so many ways in which you are exceptional, our biggest concern is whether the data you are collecting is irrational enough.

HILLARY: Sometimes when we look for that which is "the other," we base it on that which we have the least familiarity with. I think that what you are looking at may not be irrational enough.

BRAD: Sometimes what appears on the surface to be the weirdest thing you can find is really just the same old bullshit. It ends up being nothing more than the same old thing that is only wearing a different color. When you get down to it, it's just more bored people doing things to try to be interesting.

HILLARY: In other words, your data turns out to be more people who are full of you know what. The real challenge for you and what we are most concerned about concerns how to get you the kind of data that's truly going to be irrational. It needs to set your imagination on fire. The irrational part of you can then get into a dialogue with this other rational part of you that is so well-rehearsed.

REBECCA: That makes a lot of sense.

LENA: It does.

BRAD: What if you created a Facebook page entirely made up of imaginary friends on it? Or what if you fabricated an entire community of people who hang out where you live, including imaginary teachers and parents who then complain about those people? Just imagine all the gossip and talk about this group of people who don't really exist. [Rebecca laughs]

HILLARY: Maybe you could say that overnight they painted graffiti on a building, but then by morning they had removed it. Just weird stuff like that. Or you could create rumors that are like fantasy-fiction, like a virtual group or virtual gang who is doing weird stuff in your town, with virtual people complaining about it, with virtual campaigns to stop it. Now that would be extremely irrational.

REBECCA: That would take a long time and that would be cool. I've got plenty of time to do that.

BRAD: This might make you famous. That would be amazing. The trick is that you can't let anyone know because it has to really come to life. This is taking something that's dead and bringing it to life. You would become a magical woman. It would be such an amazing social experiment that even if you got the worst grades in high school, but pulled this off, you'd still get a scholarship to Harvard. [Rebecca laughs] There might be no end to the realities you invent. Your virtual people might eat stuff no one else eats, or listen to music no one else has ever heard.

REBECCA: I could invent a whole new musical genre just for the imaginary people to listen to.

BRAD: You could even use source material from your own home life. For instance, maybe they like to take camping expeditions in 60 below zero weather.

REBECCA: Yes, they love to take water samples! [Lena and Rebecca laugh]

HILLARY: You are just too bright, creative, and exceptional to have stupid data. And you're also too bright and creative to get too hung up on the bullshit that other moms and daughters get hung up on. Moms and dads will always drive you crazy—they are always going to tell you stuff you already know and get on your nerves because that's their job. You just need to do something big, something that uses more of who you are. That's what we think.

BRAD: You may not have heard the story about how another person, who also didn't believe in religion, did an experiment. He was a science fiction writer and he made up a religion just for the hell of it. Now it's a presumed religion with many followers and buildings all over the world. It was completely made up by this guy. Now I'm not saying you should create a suspect religion. I'm saying that the freedom from being attached to whether it needs to be—believable or not—gives you creative liberty to experiment with these characters, so there will be something about them that will touch the imaginations of people. As you know, whenever people talk about things in the liminal borders—things that may or may not exist in concrete reality—it feeds people's imaginations and awakens parts of human beings' experiences and allows people to enter domains they otherwise wouldn't be able to. It's the same with poetry, music, and all the rest of the creative arts.

HILLARY: I have a question for you: Have you ever had an interest in fairies?

REBECCA: Yes! Totally. [Visibly excited, Rebecca turns to Lena] Oh my God, do you care to explain that to them? Tell them about when I was really little.

LENA: [Smiling] You go ahead.

REBECCA: When I was really little we used to go camping, and we would go fairy hunting all the time in the woods and make little fairy houses and things. We were quite the little fairy experts.

LENA: My mom and dad built a big house in the country and my dad planted an apple orchard. When my mom died we buried her on the property. There was a very big tree with a large hollow in the trunk, and we would always take Rebecca to the tree so that she could look inside it to search for fairies. There was a perfect little door-shape in the tree. We would go and knock on the door to see if any fairies would answer.

REBECCA: I was quite the fairy person.

LENA: Only Rebecca could access the door in the tree, because it was so small.

REBECCA: We would leave treats near the tree and pictures for the fairies. [Brad starts playing music that fits a fairy tale, matching the excitement in the room. He continues playing as Hillary speaks]

HILLARY: Do you know what this means? The virtual society you are going to make up must have something to do with fairies, because this is an expertise you have in your life. [Brad sings a response: "The fairies say yes"] You see, everything that happens to you prepares you for the next thing, whether you believe it or not. [Brad sings: "Fairy dust everywhere] You came into this world through an exceptional birth and you were seen as exceptional by people in a faraway land, people at school, and your family notices as well. [Brad sings: They fairies saw it too] All of this has been building a stage for you to perform a grand experiment that draws upon everything that has happened to you in your life. [Brad: Fairy story, fairy world, all is fair in their air] Amazing!

REBECCA: I have always wanted to do something weird in my room, like in the movies where people try to track down some kind of big conspiracy. They put up all sorts of pictures and notes on the wall and connect everything with string. I've always wanted to do that in my room—even make a giant web. I can do that.

HILLARY: I have something for you. Close your eyes until I return. [Hillary goes into the other room and brings out an old copy of a rare book on fairies, which includes various legends and illustrations. She places it in Rebecca's lap.] You can open your eyes now because the fairies are here. I've had this book for a very long time. It was published in 1931. It's a book that has some magic and dust inside. You can feel it when you hold it. It's called *The Green Fairy Book*. Every once in a while, I take it out. I think it's a book that's been waiting for you.

REBECCA: Really? Oh my gosh. [Rebecca carefully opens and looks through the book]

BRAD: Yes. I just want to know if you are willing to make a commitment to doing this project?

REBECCA: If I can do it entirely in my own way.

HILLARY: Of course, there can be no other way. Shake on it? [Hillary leans forward and shakes Rebecca's hand]

REBECCA: I have to think about all of this. I already have lots of ideas about things I want to do. There are pictures I want to put up and strings and other things I want to glue and make. [Turns to

Lena] There are going to be lots of trips to Hobby Lobby. This is one of my skills—I can make things happen.

LENA: That's so true. She can manifest anything. As soon as she has an idea, right away she can just bring it into reality. I've never seen anything like it before.

HILLARY: That's because she has fairy mojo. [Brad sings: Fairy mojo, fairy time, fairy party all the time]

REBECCA: [Rebecca smiles] I'll get an idea in the morning, and then I'll get home and start it right away. In a week I will have transformed my room and created some huge project.

HILLARY: Your town has no idea what's coming.

LENA: [Laughing] They have no idea what's been unleashed!

REBECCA: When I write my autobiography, I can include the part about what got unleashed as a result of my coming to New Orleans.

HILLARY: Your town needs a good dose of irrationality.

LENA: [Looking at the green fairy book] Rebecca wanted a DSM-5 for her birthday, but this is a nice alternative.

HILLARY: Yes. Instead she got a book that's a lot older and wiser than the DSM-5.

BRAD: Wouldn't it be wild, if in a few months from now, you're sitting in a coffee shop and you overhear people talking about the characters you created, saying something like, "Have you heard about those people?"

REBECCA: Yes, "Have you heard what they eat?" [Rebecca giggles]

HILLARY: Sometimes you can interlace the fictional reality with real life things you do. You could get really tiny envelopes that invite people to meet in the woods, but they have to dream the meeting time. All of a sudden, you'll start hearing people say, "Hey, did you get one of those tiny envelopes?"

REBECCA: Then I'd get my own TV show someday.

BRAD: The thing is, everyone in this room knows that's possible, because you're amazing.

REBECCA: I have to get started. I have to write everything all out and plan it. It's going to take a long time, but I'm going to do it very carefully.

HILLARY: This project aims to make history—it's even bigger than you. It's an experiment in how imagination and creativity can bring forth imagination and creativity in others, liberating them from the very same problem that you've had—boredom. No one needs the DSM-5. Everyone just needs one diagnosis: boredom.

REBECCA: That's right, everyone is just very bored!

HILLARY: Every part of your life has been amazing. What happened is that you've just been in a little time out zone, waiting for your next entrance into the next chapter of amazingness.

REBECCA: The book of amazingness.

HILLARY: Yes, and now you're ready to start the next chapter. You're ready for the next entrance. You had to come to New Orleans to discover the next chapter of irrationality, the chapter that will have you creating a whole new world.

REBECCA: [Turns to Lena] You are going to have to accept things better. Be more of a cool mom. If I could come to you and tell you more of the things happening in my life without you getting all upset, then I could come to you and tell you things.

LENA: Okay. I can't wait!

[Rebecca starts teasing her mother, making a funny sound of a mother nagging. They both laugh]

HILLARY: You're going to be busy. People will think you disappeared.

BRAD: You might have to have a 'top secret' sign on your bedroom door.

REBECCA: Authorized personnel only! [She laughs]

BRAD: You have to say to your imagination, "be free," because that will help set in motion the deepest parts of your imagination.

LENA: Just like her physical birth took a long time, it's as if the birth of her imagination also has been a long time coming. It was dormant and now it's being birthed again.

HILLARY: Rebecca, you're becoming an expert at birth.

REBECCA: [To Lena] I don't even think you can imagine the magnitude of what I'm going to do. It's going to be so cool!

HILLARY: Off you go!

We received a call the next day from Lena and Rebecca. After leaving our session, they purchased a special print from a gallery in the French Quarter—a whimsical painting of a girl who looks like a fairy pulling a dragon. It turned out that the artist happened to be in the store, so they had her sign it for them. After they left the store, they discovered actor Will Ferrell shooting a scene for a movie on a street nearby. The crew asked some of the bystanders to be in the background of the shot, which of course included Rebecca and Lena. When the filming was completed, Rebecca asked Mr. Ferrell to sign the print they just purchased. What he wrote was quite apt for the situation: "For Rebecca: To happy accidents and joyous circumstances—may your path inspire others!"

Budding creative therapists should be aware that Mohandas K. Gandhi entitled his autobiography, *The Story of My Experiments with Truth*. Why not name the next chapter of your life (which begins today) as, "The Story of My Experiments with Creative Therapy?" Like Rebecca, conduct an innovative experiment. If you want, perform talking to a therapy fairy or if you prefer, hum along with a singing dairy cow. After all, Carl Whitaker was from Wisconsin amidst the dairy farms. Also, feel free to write a letter to Gandhi, but write it in the air without any ink or paper. After all, you are addressing the unseen. Remember that the mist of mystery is found in what is deeply felt as the heart ventures into the creative steam of a dream stream.

Imagine that you and every other therapist on the planet have sessions that may oscillate between the old world of "boredom" and the unexplored frontier of "oredom." Without the treasures and gold found in life's ore, you too easily get bored. Creatively experiment with boredom and see what catches your interest, even if it is the tiniest of sparks. Follow its lead to oredom, the kingdom of the ore holding transformational gold. Learn how to further tinker with boredom in order to avoid a relapse into creative paralysis. Do it to write an ongoing therapy autobiography about experimental adventures that seek the big room of yet to be found mystery.

Consider getting a diary to write down the results of all the prescriptions assigned in this book. Recognize how they offer experiments with you. If you wish, call this a "Fairy Tale Book," your account of tinkering with therapy life. Come to appreciate that this is like sprinkling fairy dust that brings enchantment and wonder to all. We actually refer to our own creative therapy work as a "project for the creation of live fairy tales." When mystery and its gifts come through the creative therapy birth canal, we express our heartfelt celebration. Did you know that you are also a teaching and fairy tale waiting to be born? Let's start celebrating because, with this recognition and jubilation, rebirth begins.

Recognize that you can transform a writing pen into a magic wand or a computer keyboard into an alchemical skeleton key. With them better incantations and nonclinical fairy tales can arise as you keep a record of the experiments that go past the containment of former therapy. Be less therapeutic and more healing. Become a facilitator of mystery and mess less with misery.

One more thing: after we opened the door for the mother and daughter to leave, Hillary said, "Come back. We almost forgot. You need to be costumed." They came back to rummage through Hillary's costume wardrobe and were outfitted in crazy hats, feather boas, and wigs. Then they were sent on their way, laughing together as they walked down the street. You, too, should not head into your next session without making some kind of costume change. Perhaps a bit of dust sprinkled on your shoe or a hair from a beard or the crumb of some pie for the top of your head?

6

THE LADY WITH TWO VIOLINS

The following are transcriptions of two healing sessions conducted with a sixty-year-old woman named Lenke. The first session was held in front of an audience in Budapest, Hungary, and the second was held privately three weeks later. We were joined in both sessions by Dr. Dezsoe Birkas, who had been Lenke's therapist.

HILLARY: Thank you for coming. Please share with us whatever you would like.

LENKE: I have a problem. I only have enough strength to get the basic, important things done in my everyday life, and after that I feel tired. At one point I felt like I didn't want to live, as if I couldn't get up in the morning because there was nothing to live for. I got over the worst of that with the help of my therapist. But still, I no longer have the kind of life force that I used to have. My creativity and any sense of free-flowing experience are blocked. When I try to take a step forward and make plans to do different things in my life, I always feel a resistance. It feels like a kind of negative energy arises. Therefore, I don't dare to really live fully. I'm in a sort of vegetative state. I feel aimless and listless. This is what I would like to change. I am a believer, but my prayers don't show me the way out. I'm an older woman, but still the time ahead of me is too long to just count the days and be content knowing that most of my life has passed. Also, there are many struggles in my workplace. I feel hindered. I'm right at the age when I can retire. I'd like to put down my profession because I am much more interested in other things. I'm an accountant.

I cannot plan my private life because of my job. My daily struggles at work take away my strength. I have a daughter and a little granddaughter who bring happiness to my life, but very often my discussions with my daughter are about their needs, never about mine. I have to give all the time. I do this voluntarily, but I'm like a servant in the family and in my workplace and so joy eludes me.

DEZSOE: [After a long pause] Lenke used to play the violin.

LENKE: [She smiles a little at Dezsoe] I haven't played in a very long time. I took my violin out of the closet not too long ago and it completely fell apart. It was like taking something out of a coffin like a dead body. But I purchased another one. The other one has a nice sound.

BRAD: So you have two violins: One is for the you that is very tired, and the other one is for the you that wants to play and hear the music again. I have one question: Have you ever prayed while playing the violin? You mentioned that you pray, but we want to know whether you have prayed with your violin.

LENKE: No.

BRAD: I think that is what's missing.

LENKE: It's difficult because I have not played for such a long time.

BRAD: It doesn't matter.

HILLARY: Even if you play only two notes. We recently had a session with a famous Hungarian musician. During our session he composed a song with just two notes. We discussed how all he needed were those two notes to get his life started again in the direction that he wanted. It actually only takes one note.

BRAD: Yes, it's better to play one single note and make it a new kind of musical prayer that expresses its sound with all your heart, body, and soul. You can do it with your violin.

LENKE: It's difficult to put into words what I am asking for.

BRAD: That's why you need a musical note to say it better. Without the musical prayer in your life, the words and life itself get stuck. Where would you do this? Is there a room in your house that you would choose to play the violin while making a musical prayer?

LENKE: I live alone, so it doesn't matter where I do it.

BRAD: The bedroom? The living room? In front of the window?

LENKE: [Chuckles] No, not in front of the window.

HILLARY: The closet?

LENKE: [Laughs] No. I could use any room. The problem is I live in an apartment, so I have to be careful about noise, although the man above me plays the guitar and drums.

BRAD: You could also do it in the park if you want. It's up to you. I just wonder where you will decide to do it the first time. The first time you do it should be in a very special place. If the things you tell us about your life are serious—that you really feel stuck and want more creativity to come forth, then you will do this. If it is true that you want the important things in your life to come back, that you really want the energy to flow, and if you really do have two violins, then for the first time in your life you need to make a musical note with the violin and musically pray at the same time, doing so as if your life depends on it. You are lucky because you have two violins. If you only had the old one, you would have a problem. But because you have two, you have an opportunity for a second life. The violin needs to come back to life, along with you, along with your musical prayer, the heartfelt note, and everything else.

[Dezsoe turns to Lenke and says something to her in Hungarian. She chuckles and nods]

DEZSOE: I asked her if I could share something with you. Her mother has sent her several postcards with a picture of a violin and a rose on them. There is an old Hungarian song about a violin and a rose. When Lenke told me about the postcards from her mother, I was reminded of that song and sang it to her.

BRAD: [To Lenke] You are very lucky. The ancestral composers and musicians of the past are using many people to bring you the same message: your mother, your therapist, and us.

HILLARY: And your violin.

BRAD: [Brad reaches out and takes hold of Lenke's hand. He has a vibration in his voice and trembles her hand as he speaks] It's time you listened to the special musical message coming to you. You are being offered a second life with a second violin. If you want that life, it doesn't matter how you feel right now or tonight or tomorrow. If you really want that second life you have to pick up that second violin. Do it in spite of how you feel. Don't even do it for you. Do it for the violin. Do it for that Hungarian song or do it for Franz Liszt or Amadeus Mozart or Ludwig Beethoven. Do it for the rose on the postcard. And then watch what happens. [Dezsoe is visibly moved by these words and takes a deep, audible breath] Do it for Dezsoe. Do it for us. Do it for your grandchildren, your children, your whole family, and the musician upstairs. One evening that musician will hear a single violin note as a prayer. Even if he just barely hears a tone, it may be enough to change his music. Then a child outside might hear him drum and play the guitar in a way that changes his life.

That child might then start running through the park in a way that surprises a bird flying overhead who then catches a new song. Somewhere, someone will hear that bird sing a different song and on that same day, that person will decide to open her closet and she too will take out an old instrument and bring it back to life. This is your comeback coming through. Reach for that violin. Hold it in your arms. It wants your heart to give it attention. It needs your arms; it needs your movement. There is a secret seldom told—and no one knows whether it's only partially true or wholly true—but sometimes the Creator of the universe gets tired trying to take care of all the prayers. Music is needed to make the world strong. Let that work be done through your hands. As I once heard my grandparents say to me, God's hands work through others and this includes music. Make the sound that is the new prayer … That violin is waiting for you.

[There is a long pause and the room is silent. What Lenke doesn't know is that two days prior to her coming we held a session with one of the seminar participants in which we helped him discover that he could make a deep, healing tone with his voice. Since that session, whenever the creative therapy temperature rose in other sessions we asked this young man to make that tone for the client. It naturally resulted that the entire audience would also join him in singing the uplifting tone. Brad now turns to the audience and asks them to make this sound]

BRAD: Now I need everyone to offer a musical tone. Make that healing sound that comes from your heart.

[The audience begins to sing various tones in harmony, led by the young man. Lenke closes her eyes. Hillary stands and lays her vibrating hands on Lenke's head while Brad sends a vibration through her hand. This goes on for several minutes, then Brad claps loudly once and the singing stops. Lenke opens her eyes and looks at Brad, who smiles at her]

BRAD: There is a light coming from you. I can see it. That's what your violin has been waiting for. This is what the world has been waiting for. It's what you have been waiting for.

LENKE: [Wiping tears from her eyes and smiling] Thank you. Yes.

HILLARY: So will you play your violin tonight?

LENKE: Yes, this evening.

BRAD: Very good. It's time to come back to life.

[Lenke, Brad, and Hillary stand and embrace]

Roughly one week after Lenke's session we held a two-day public event in Budapest. Lenke was in attendance. During the second day when the creative therapy temperature was high, Brad placed his hands again on Lenke's head and discovered that she had a wonderful somatic vibration. He told her this and we celebrated her special vibration in front of the audience. One week after the service, Lenke returned for the following session:

BRAD: So, how are the violins doing?

LENKE: They are fine. I see the way forward. The vibrations keep moving in me. I still think I need to practice the violin more. One big breakthrough that happened is that I have started crying again. For quite a long time I was not able to cry—it got stuck inside me and wouldn't come out. But recently, when things became very difficult at work I was able to cry about it. It was a relief for me. That means a lot to me, because I used to cry a lot. I suffered a lot lately for not being able to cry. [Lenke takes a long pause] I was thinking of telling you today about the point at which my life broke in two pieces. I would like to understand this more in a spiritual way. Not to understand it more in the usual way, but to re-evaluate this from a spiritual perspective.

As a child I grew up as a believer, as a Christian. We had a neighbor who was a medical doctor. He was also a believer. He had studied in China and practiced natural Chinese healing methods. As a child I witnessed him do many interesting and miraculous healings. My father was healed by this man after other doctors had told him that there was no chance of recovery. My worldview was shaped by that experience and I became a more open person as a result. Instead of studying music, however, I studied mathematics. During my university years, I got to know many students from abroad who studied in Hungary. I made many friends from around the world. I fell in love with a man from northern Africa. He was the man who I loved most in my life. He loved me too, and my family accepted him. I got pregnant by him when I was 22. We decided to marry. I thought of going to Africa with him. He was Muslim, but not very religious. He feared God, however, and accepted my Christianity. One summer, during break, he went home to Africa and did not return for quite a long time. My belly continued to grow. Then one day he returned to Hungary and told me that his family would not allow him to marry a European Christian woman because they had already arranged his marriage. He would not dare challenge his family. Two or three weeks went by and we were ground down by this decision. He wished to stay by my side, but it was very difficult. Then one day I started to have pain and I went to the hospital. They tried to help me but there were additional complications and my child was born very prematurely. When she was born I could not dare to look at her because I was afraid she would die. They took her to another hospital where they have a center for premature babies. [Lenke begins to weep] In three days they sent a telegram to me that she had died. I never saw her.

The nurse gave me an injection, and ever since then I have had an illness. The boy decided to challenge his family and stay with me, but we were both too broken. We tried to fight for our relationship for another couple years. I then became afraid because he told me that if the same complication with our baby were to have happened in Africa, I probably would have died because they don't have good medical care where he lives. I became afraid of the thought of living in Africa with him. I then began to think that perhaps someone had put a curse on me. I became very sick and I couldn't eat or sleep. I was dizzy all the time. I was given some medicine, but no psychotherapy. I went from doctor to doctor, but they only tranquilized me. There came a time when I could not even walk along the street. I finished university with one year of delay and I had to decide whether I would go to Africa with him or stay here. I brooded over the decision, but in the end, I decided to stay in Hungary. There was something in me that told me that I had to stay. The boy went back to Africa. It was a very difficult time, because later on when I would walk along the street and see an African man, I would think to myself, "He is coming for me." Eventually he married an African woman. Sometimes we still exchange letters. He sends me photos of his family. This relationship is still an affectionate one.

I have thought quite a lot about this over the years and tried to understand what forces were behind these events in my life. Thirty-eight years have gone by since then and I still see a therapist. I really thought that I was cursed and that I would never manage to recover, but I also think there must have been another force—Christ—holding me. I have always felt that it was Jesus who did not allow me to leave Hungary because it would have meant death for me. Later I gave birth to a daughter who is now an adult. Her father is not a believer, but he was open to alternative medicine. We had a doctor who tried to heal us both through those means, but my husband was against Jesus and strong faith. When my daughter became sick I decided to christen her, because one night my daughter spontaneously began to pray in her bed, and then she did so every evening after that.

My husband did not come to the christening ceremony, and then slowly we grew apart and separated. I brought up my daughter on my own. She met a boy who is now her husband. He studies theology. Over the years I maintained my interest in alternative healing such as spontaneous healing and energy medicine. I felt I had this inside me, so I studied it. I used it for healing or the alleviation of pain for myself and for my daughter. When my daughter's husband started his theology studies, she then turned against it and told me that it was not a good thing. I learned that you are not supposed to say that you do energy healing in front of our Protestant congregation. But I see that they are both one. I see my Christian faith and energy medicine as one. So, I live in this dual reality: I go to church and listen to the preaching and yet I miss spirituality very much. [Brad and Hillary recognize what Lenke is saying about her spiritual life. They smile and clap, as Brad grabs Lenke's hand and spontaneously lets out a loud shrieking sound that is often heard in southern Africa among Bushman healers. Lenke nods and smiles at this celebration]

BRAD: I must say, this is such a wonderful story even though it is filled with great suffering. Remember that we told everyone at the healing service that you have a special vibration. I told Hillary that same night: "I cannot believe her vibration. It is just perfect." We both agreed, and I wondered, "Why does she have this amazing vibration?" We kept discussing it and asking each other, "I wonder if she is playing that violin? I wonder why she has such a wonderful vibration?" And now we know why. Now we know so many things happened to you to make your life a spiritual journey. The only way you can have a vibration like yours is to receive that kind of suffering that breaks the heart. Without a broken heart the body is unable to receive this vibration.

[Brad gets a vibration in his voice, and speaks slowly and softly, sometimes singing as his speech becomes more melodic] Just watching that healer you lived next to as a child and being near him was enough to start something inside of you, including the deep knowing of its truth. Your faith has always held you even when you felt uncertain. You are still here, and you have that vibration. Curses are like a sneeze—they involve a lot of air. You have something that's even harder to receive. The curse you received was a true heartbreak that also brought a blessing. The suffering of love has made you soft and open to something otherwise unfelt. That's what made you a person who could have the vibration that we immediately recognized. Thank you for letting us know who you really are.

Even through all the disappointments, the contradictions, the dualisms, the tensions, the unfairness, and the loneliness, in spite of all that, here you are. Here you are with the suffering that made you soft and opened your heart. When your heart was broken it was opened for God to pour love into you, the vibration inside of you.

Nothing you said really surprised us. At the same time, I'm shocked to be holding the hand of someone so touched who is also so humble. You're not sick. Even when you're sick, you're not sick. You're not weak. Even when you feel weak, you're not weak. I'm going to tell you something now: The only thing wrong with you is that your vibration is right. Listen to and feel the truth of this vibration. It's so important to musically pray with that note on the violin because it honors the vibration. It is the same vibration. Stop thinking you need to practice. You have a perfect vibration. Nothing else matters now. Play the violin. As long as you have that vibration, that single note will become a holy musical prayer. It's time you stopped doubting your natural gifts. It's time for you to step into elder wisdom.

For people like you, it is always the case that you think you have always been wrong, until you get older and then you realize that you were always right. If you had known all of this when you were younger you wouldn't have ripened and matured. Now is the time to know you're right and to see all those preachers and ministers and doctors as being lost in the dark. The heart that hasn't been broken is only a heart that has been hardened. Welcome to being an elder.

I don't want to ever hear you say, "I need to practice." I don't ever want to hear you say, "I need a doctor." I don't ever want to hear you say, "I don't understand." That is the talk of someone who has not become an elder. You are now an elder who lived all those years with all that heartbreak, who is now waking up to find that you have everything that is important—this vibration of your body must meet the violin's vibrating string.

[Brad gets a stronger vibration in his voice as he says an old-fashioned prayer like he would in a healing ceremony, something she earlier requested outside the room. Seated in his chair, he leans forward and places one hand on Lenke's head]

So, we bless you in the name of all that is holy.
Bless this child who became a woman
and carried a child,
who carried the suffering.
Now is the time for her to come into elderhood

and to hold the truth of what is left.
After all of everything that happened to her,
what is left are two violins,
and room for two words.
Sometimes the words say, "thank you,"
sometimes the words say, "praise God,"
sometimes the words say, "I do,"
"I am,"
"I'm yours."

So, we ask this blessing today, which we are going to call graduation day.

We grant through the musical prayer bestowed upon us, this holy diploma marked upon you. [Brad makes a spiritual symbol on Lenke's forehead] You formerly bore the suffering,
Now you have graduated.
Even though the road, string, and song are easy to forget,
You are always on it.
So, use that heart and use those hands,
And all the words, notes, and vibrations that come to you.

[Brad rises from his chair and walks over to the piano and begins playing an old sacred song. Hillary stands and places her vibrating hands on Lenke's head. Brad's music changes to simple chords as he sings the following words:]

We take your words that you shared with us as a sacred offering.
You who have loved; you who have loved.
You have been opened in the deepest way,
Placed in the darkest of dark, in the loneliest place.
In the darkest place is made room for the brightest light.
In the most difficult suffering is made room for the greatest spiritual joy.
This is how it has always been.
There are no shortcuts and no easy way.
But you have made it to graduation day.
Time for you to go into the world
As the light that illumines the dark,
As the joyful heart whose violin is ready to play.
May your life vibrate the way you already do.
You already knew but were too humble to let yourself know.
All we did was mirror your truth.
We saw, and we felt something holy about you.
We thank you for coming into our lives.
We, like you, have had our hearts broken.
We, like you, have been broken into thousands of pieces before.

But we were put back together by a musical mystery just like you.
Happy graduation day.
It's still going to hurt from time to time.
You're still going to suffer.
You're still going to remember the pain.
You're still going to trip and fall.
But now, for the first time in your life
You deeply know that you have a violin.
You actually have two.
One you just repaired, just like you have been repaired.
The other is just waiting,
Like you have been waiting.
Both broken and both made whole.
This is you.
You are both the violins.
Let God play your life.
The next time we see you, we better see a violin in your hands.

[Brad brings his music to a close. Lenke slowly opens her eyes and comes back from her trance. Hillary and Lenke embrace, Brad and Lenke embrace, as the session concludes]

Creative change only requires a single tone to express its pulse of life. You must be tuned, transformed, and then played by something bigger than a conscious tactic, memorized routine, or a no longer creative line. Life must play the therapy string that attaches you to the source and force of change. We invite you to imagine that an invisible violin sits in your closet waiting for you to find it. As soon as you can, go to your closest and pretend to find this lost violin that is invisible except to the eyes of imagination. Rest the base of this unseen violin on your shoulder and imagine playing one perfectly inspired tone, yielding a vibration heard all round the world. Hear it in your inner performance room. As your hand holds the bow and crosses the string, your creative life awakens as the vibration is felt.

The Caribbean shakers, like the earlier Shakers and Quakers, sometimes receive imaginary musical instruments in their dreams. They know that all kinds of musical mysteries can take place upon unconscious concert ground. After a follow-up session with us, her therapist reported this outcome: "She played her violin in an effortless and improvisational way whilst praying. The atmosphere exploded and ever since she desires to do nothing else! She felt well for the first time in 30 years!"

When Lenke plays her violin, she is playing not only for herself, but for all creative therapists as well. In the same way that the flapping wings of a butterfly in Asia are complexly connected to the taste of ice cream that a child experiences in Idaho, the heated spiritual atmosphere of a violinist's prayer can send a vibration to the string of your imagined violin. In this shared resonance, you become inseparable from her musical prayer. Imagine this as you play a single note and make the kind of musical prayer a traditional healer from any spiritual tradition might voice. Lenke is doing the same, along with others throughout the world. In this noteworthy way, the creative therapist can move from a solo violin to a duet, trio, quartet, and symphonic orchestra that fills the world with joyful sound. Edmond de Goncourt reminds us that like a poet, each of us "puts up a ladder to a star and climbs it while playing a violin." As your uplifting musical note enables you to rise, know that pies are coming out of fairy ovens, warming hearts everywhere as a previously unheard mystery prevails over all ails.

7

BUILDING A HOUSE FOR A GENTLE FEATHER

The following two sessions were conducted in Budapest, Hungary with an older man named, Tamás. The first session took place in front of an audience and the second took place privately one month later.

BRAD: It is nice to meet you, thank you for coming.

TAMÁS: Thank you for the opportunity.

HILLARY: Please share with us whatever you would like to share—anything at all.

BRAD: Even something you had not planned to talk about. Perhaps something you have never talked about in your whole life. Anything.

TAMÁS: Well, in this moment there are not many things that come to my mind. I have some difficult circumstances in my life, but it's probably better that I don't talk about them. It concerns my father.

HILLARY: It's up to you what you'd like to share.

TAMÁS: I had a very strict father. He oppressed me very much in my childhood. He wouldn't let me grow. He had very strict principles and I was supposed to follow them, but it was not good for me. This experience followed me throughout the rest of my life in a negative way. That's it in a nutshell.

BRAD: [After a short pause] As you were speaking I had a funny image pop into my mind. It's an unusual image, a surprising image that turned into a question. In all of your many years—from the time you were a small boy, then an adolescent, then a young man, and up until now—at any point during that time, did you catch or pick up a feather?

TAMÁS: [Pauses to think] Yes.
BRAD: Did you ever keep a special feather?
TAMÁS: No.
HILLARY: So after you picked up the feather, you let it go?
TAMÁS: I kept it for a while, but not for a long time.
BRAD: That's what I am wondering about. How long did you keep it? One day? One week? How long?
TAMÁS: About a week.
HILLARY: So you remember how long you kept it.
TAMÁS: It was during my childhood.
BRAD: About how old were you?
TAMÁS: About eight or ten years old.
HILLARY: Was it a white feather or a colored feather?
TAMÁS: A white feather.
BRAD: A white feather.
TAMÁS: Yes.
BRAD: How big was it? Was it this big, or this big? [Brad shows different sizes with his hands]
TAMÁS: About this big. [Tamás uses his hands to show a feather about eight inches long]
BRAD: That's interesting. Wouldn't it be something if now in your life—maybe even tomorrow or tonight or this week—you came across that same feather?
TAMÁS: [Chuckles] I would be surprised.
HILLARY [SMILING]: That would be a surprise.
TAMÁS: Yes, it would be. It would be a big surprise.
BRAD: Yes. Wouldn't it be something if you found the same exact feather that you lost before?
TAMÁS: [Shakes his head and pauses to consider it] That would be something. I would not be able to explain it.
BRAD: I'm going to tell you a story that is impossible to believe.
TAMÁS: If it's impossible to believe, then I'm going to believe it.
BRAD: Many years ago, I dreamed of some feathers. I woke up and thought, "What is this?" The next night I dreamed again of the same feathers and I saw myself in a faraway country in the Amazon rainforest. The third night I dreamed of the same feathers again. Soon afterwards I received a phone call from an organization in Paraguay, asking me to give a speech to an audience of psychotherapists. To make a long story short, when I went there I met the Amazonian Indians who live in Paraguay and they said to me, "Here is the feather that you dreamed." That is just the beginning of the story. I thought to myself, "Wow. This is unexplainable." Shortly after I went home, and I was asked to

give a speech in New York. I decided to take the collection of feathers from the Amazon with me. The feathers were all tied to a stick of wood shaped like a "Y," sort of like a small wand. I brought the feathers to my speech and was telling the audience about the story. As I lifted up the stick, a feather flew off and floated all the way into the audience and landed on someone's lap. I thought, "I should let that person keep the feather." When I returned home the next week, I found that same feather lying on the ground at my front door. I cannot explain this. But, based on my own experience, I believe that if you found a white feather as a child and took it home and lived with it for a week, it is possible that the same white feather could come back to you.

TAMÁS: [Nodding] Yes.

BRAD: It's also possible that you could go looking for the feather. You could go find a feather that is white and the same size. It might be the same one, or it might be the brother of the feather, it might be the uncle of the feather, it might be the father of the feather, or the grandfather of the feather. When you find it, bring it home, and in a private moment, say to the feather, "I'm never letting you go." This is something you could do.

TAMÁS: There is a chance this could happen because I do take a lot of walks. My wife and I walk a lot together in town and through the parks. I live on the outskirts of the city and we walk in big open places where it is possible to find a feather.

HILLARY: If you really wanted to find a feather that is a relative of the other feather, or similar to the other feather, you could find it.

TAMÁS: Yes, I think so. I remember it—I have kept this image of the feather with me.

BRAD: Very good. This supports what we're thinking.

TAMÁS: Yes?

BRAD: I have a very strong feeling that this is very, very important for your life. You must find this feather. I feel this quite strongly because I think the first feather that came to you—the one that you spent one week with—taught you how to be soft. Without your knowing this was taking place, it taught you softness.

TAMÁS: There is something to that, yes. I usually don't talk about that. As people would say, that is not how a man should behave.

HILLARY: That's right.

TAMÁS: But here with you now, I feel free to talk about it. Otherwise, I would suggest that the feather means something different. I would not show myself in this way, but instead I would hide and behave in a way that others expect. When I think back on my work and my life, I see that my whole life was about fulfilling expectations, wearing a mask, and doing what was expected of me. This is why I was never unemployed. I had to make compromises. I had a co-worker who didn't make compromises. He came to me one day and told me he wanted to tell our boss exactly what he thought, that he didn't want to make compromises. I told him to go ahead, but be careful. In one month that man lost his job. Then he complained that he could not find a job and support his family. That's how life is, at least in Hungary.

BRAD: On the one hand, you had a very strong father who taught you—

TAMÁS: [Tamás interrupts] He was strong in a way, but in a way, he was also very weak. He had a kind of power that made me and my younger brother feel afraid of him.

BRAD: So your father could be very hard.

TAMÁS: Yes. He could be very hard.

HILLARY: On the one hand, you learned about being strong and hard, but you secretly also learned to be soft because you had a feather live with you for one week.

TAMÁS: [Chuckles and nods] Yes.

BRAD: Yes. That's an interesting secret.

TAMÁS: This is very interesting. This is a totally new way of looking at it. I never thought of it that way before.

BRAD: In many ways that feather was smart to find you because you were able to keep its secret, which is that the strongest men are secretly soft, and have been visited by a feather who lived with them for at least one week. Wouldn't it be something if there were other men around the world who also found the same white feather at the same age, and who also had tough, hard fathers? And the feather taught them to be soft in one week, which they also kept a secret? Maybe there are twelve of you in the world. Maybe twenty-five. Maybe there is one man like this in each country in the world.

TAMÁS: I have met several men who became my friends who first appeared to be very hard, but then they showed me their softness. But they only showed it in front of me because they knew they could trust me. They knew I would never use it against them.

BRAD: Of course because the feather chose you. This is what I think. I also think there are two things you need to do. First, you need to find a white feather. Then you need to make it a special home. Maybe you could build it a little house.

TAMÁS: Yes, I am a very good carpenter. I make things all the time. I like building things very much. I have all the necessary tools.

HILLARY: Would you make the feather house out of wood or out of metal?

TAMÁS: Out of wood.

BRAD: That's what I thought. What kind of wood?
TAMÁS: A softer wood.
HILLARY: Would it look like a box or would it look like a little house?
TAMÁS: I would try to make a little house.
BRAD: That's wonderful! Wow!
TAMÁS: [Smiles and laughs] Yes.
HILLARY: That feather is very lucky!
TAMÁS: The wood suggests closeness and the house provides shelter. I'm a very home-centered man, so to speak.
BRAD: Wonderful.
TAMÁS: Home is important to me. So is my family. I have tried to learn from the mistakes of my father and not repeat them. He had a different view—he took advantage of his leadership position and took advantage of the women who worked with him and had affairs. But he did not find his happiness. He divorced my mother. He was never happy. At the end of his life he told my mother, "You were my first, truest love." A person is not supposed to leave his family that way.
BRAD: Maybe, just maybe, when your father was ten years old a white feather fell in front of him, but he did not pick it up and take it home.
TAMÁS: My grandfather—his father—was a very kind man.
HILLARY: It's possible, though, that this happened.
TAMÁS: Yes.
BRAD: We can never know all the mysteries of life, but maybe all the men in your family before you, including your grandfather and your father, waited for you to pick up the feather. Maybe your father wanted to pick up the feather, but then he thought, "I'm going to wait for my son to pick it up." Wouldn't that be an interesting story?
TAMÁS: That would be very interesting, but it doesn't fit my imagination of him. He was selfish and loved himself the most, unfortunately. In his last years he started to change a little. He suffered from remorse in his last years. He told me that he couldn't look back at his life because to do so brought him suffering. I did everything differently than my father and as a result, my son became a different man. He is happy and has good self-esteem. I invested a lot of effort into him. He became a successful man, and this makes me very happy. This makes up for my relationship with my father.
HILLARY: Yes, because you carried the teaching of the feather. What is most important now is for the feather to return and for you to make it a home.

TAMÁS: Yes. I'm going to look for it. During my walks with my wife I'm going to keep an eye out for it. On the mountain, in the woods, in the park—there probably has been a feather on my path many times already but I didn't see it. From now on, I will pay attention.

BRAD: Do you have grandchildren?

TAMÁS: No.

HILLARY: Someday, perhaps?

TAMÁS: Yes, that would make me very happy! [Laughs]

BRAD: Someday in the future, after you have found the feather and made it a house, you will show that house to a child—maybe it will be your grandchild or another child who looks up to you like a grandfather. You will open it up and say, "Look at grandfather's secret. I have a feather. I found it when I was ten years old. I lived with a white feather for one week and kept it a secret. Then I found another white feather. It might be the same one, or it might be its brother or its sister or its father. I made a home for it. This feather is always going to stay in our home. It will be here for you in the future. It will be here for your children and your grandchildren. Never again will a man or a woman in our family be left alone without the teaching of a feather."

TAMÁS: [Tamás nods and begins to weep] So it will be. I will do that.

HILLARY: What a gift it is for all the generations of your family to be able to receive the secret of your good life. It's wonderful. Thank you for being such a big man who is both strong and soft, whose secret friend is a white feather.

TAMÁS: [Tamás is visibly moved] Thank you. Thank you very, very much. I will take this moment—this day—and keep it with me for my whole life. This had a deep, deep effect on me. I thank you so much.

BRAD: Thank you. You have brought teaching to all of us.

TAMÁS: [Wiping his eyes and shaking his head as if in disbelief] I thank you. I received a teaching today that is unbelievable for me. It is never too late for something new to arise.

BRAD: The feather is waiting to be found and for you to bring it home and make it a home. Can you take a photograph of the house you build and send it to us?

TAMÁS: Of course.

HILLARY: Wonderful. We will put it on our desk.

TAMÁS: You honor me.

BRAD: This is wonderful.

HILLARY: It is a gift for us.

TAMÁS: Thank you. Thank you so much.

[Brad, Tamás, and Hillary rise and embrace]

One month later, we received a phone call from Tamás's therapist who told us that since our last session he had again become very depressed and was having a difficult time. We asked if he would like to have another session with us and he accepted. When Tamás entered the room, he and Brad embrace.

BRAD: It is very good to see you.

TAMÁS: I am very happy that you and your dear wife are still here in Budapest, and that we can meet again. Unfortunately, I have had a hard time. I felt very good when I left the session with you last time. I felt as if everything was good and that I no longer had any depression. But after that, I had a relapse of my depression. Somehow it just came on and I could not fight it off. I was very active, but now I'm physically exhausted. It is difficult for me to get up in the morning. I am often in a panic, I am tense, and I feel afraid of the future. I am afraid of becoming crazy. On the one hand, I can't be active and want to lie down all the time, but whenever I lie down crazy thoughts come to me. [Tamás begins to cry] The last time I was here it was like a feast. I felt so good. It was so extraordinary.

BRAD: How far did you get with the tasks?

TAMÁS: I found the feather and I have made parts of the house. I should assemble them, but I'm unable to do anything. I can't concentrate. It's very difficult. I find it very hard to go on and to carry on with my day-to-day activities. I feel weak. I feel like I'm being ground up in a mill. Some people in my current state would go to the mental hospital, but I don't want to go there. I hate those places; they are terrible.

HILLARY: How far did you get with the house? Did you pick out the pieces of wood?

TAMÁS: The walls have been cut, but the roof has not been made. One side of the house will be made of glass or translucent plastic.

HILLARY: Wow! That sounds amazing. [Brad nods in agreement]

TAMÁS: The feather will stand inside the house. I will drill a hole in the middle, and the feather will stand inside it. One wall will be translucent so that you can see the feather inside.

BRAD: I think nothing should stop you from making that house. Not even the worst depression should stop you, as difficult as that might be to hear. If I could look into the future and tell you, "I can't explain how I know this, but if you make this house it will save the life of a child," then I think you would finish that house no matter how badly you feel. If you knew building the house would save a child's life, you would do it no matter what, am I right?

TAMÁS: Yes. That would give me the necessary strength.

BRAD: Because you know that when something is important enough, you can do it. It doesn't matter if you have to crawl across the floor or drink extra coffee and stay up all night. Building this feather house is one of those important things. I actually think it's possible that someone's life will be affected based on whether or not you finish this house in a timely manner. It might even be the child inside of you, wanting to be released.

TAMÁS: I have been living in a prison for a very long time. This thing has affected my life for a long time, ever since I was a child, because of the way my father treated me emotionally. He only started to change a little when he was very old, toward the end of his life.

HILLARY: If you had to finish this house because you knew it was a life and death matter, how long would it take you?

TAMÁS: Probably two days, but it requires so much precision and patience that I don't have right now. Not long ago my son asked me to make something with wood that required even more precision than this house and I was able to finish it. It required a lot of patience. I was happy with the amount of patience I had to finish it. I always thought while making it how good it was that I was not depressed. I was free of depression for years after I started working with my therapist. I thought that this would continue, but then I had a conflict with the wife of my father after he died. Ever since then, I cannot find my way out of the depression. This woman is very strong. We had a conflict.

BRAD: It sounds like she put a curse on you.

TAMÁS: I haven't visited her for quite a long time after my father died because whenever I went to see her, she would always find a way to hurt or criticize me. Nothing I did was good enough. Nothing I said was good enough. She was sometimes like that even before the death of my father.

BRAD: It's amazing that she has such a strong effect on you.

TAMÁS: I haven't seen her for quite a while but, yes, somehow it seems possible that she put a curse on me.

BRAD: I have known people who thought they had a curse. They really believed they had a curse.

TAMÁS: I don't think that she would curse me on purpose. It was just that nothing I did was ever good enough. For example, one time I shoveled some snow for her. I broke up the ice on her sidewalk, and there was just a tiny piece of ice left. When she came outside she started pointing at it and criticizing me, saying, "Look at that! What did you do?" I think it hurts me that she behaves that way. There was a time when she told me that I was one of the people in her life she liked the most, second only to my father. When my depression first came back I had a traffic accident and I had to wait three years for the trial. I only received a fine, but I was constantly agonizing about it during those three years.

BRAD: May I say something? Whether this woman knows it or not, she found the perfect way to mess with your life, perhaps the perfect way to accidentally given you a curse. It is because you are a perfectionist. Unless you can do a job perfectly, you probably won't do it.

TAMÁS: [Nodding] Yes, that's right.

BRAD: When you shoveled the snow, I know it was perfect. But when someone who you think loves and respects you then criticizes it and says it's terrible and points out some flaw, this really messes with your mind. Such a thing wouldn't bother others, but it would really mess with you.

TAMÁS: [Nodding] Yes, that's exactly the way it is.

BRAD: Actually, I don't think you're depressed. I think you received an accidental curse. Such a curse feels terrible. It makes you feel like sometimes you want to go to the hospital. [Tamás nods] I once had a client who was a famous professional football player in the United States. He was a huge, very large man. He was very tough, but there was a woman in his life who he said put a curse on him. Everyone told him that it was ridiculous for him to believe this. He ended up in the hospital where they diagnosed him as being depressed and schizophrenic. He struggled greatly until he could break the curse. He was a very famous American sports star. When he came to me and I heard his story I told him, "You are not depressed, and you are not schizophrenic. You are cursed." He replied, "Yes, I think I am cursed, and I know the woman who did it." It was his ex-wife. After they divorced he remarried, and his ex-wife then said to him, "I'll get you." After that, he worried about it all the time. I asked him, "Do you still have the same furniture in your new bedroom that you had with your ex-wife?" He said, "Yes, it was the same furniture." I immediately exclaimed, "Are you crazy? That's how you're cursed. You can't sleep with the same furniture that you had with your ex-wife. Throw it away. Go home tonight and burn it." He responded, "Oh, I can't. The furniture is too nice." I said, "Are you crazy? If you burn it, I promise you will be free." He told me there was no way he would do that because the furniture was too nice. So, I said, "Can you chop off one leg of a cabinet and burn it?"

He said, "No, that's too much." I talked to him for one hour until he finally agreed that he would cut one tiny piece of the bedroom lampshade off and burn it in the front yard. When he did that, the curse was over. He was so happy that he then got rid of all the furniture. So, when you tell me that this woman who trusts, loves, and respects you and who knows you are a perfectionist criticizes your perfectly done job, I can easily see the impact that would have. It's the same as giving you a curse because it makes you doubt everything and doubt yourself. Such a thing makes you wonder whether she sees something about you that you never saw before, and that feeling starts to grow and run away with itself.

HILLARY: A curse only needs to be like a tiny seed that is planted. Once it is there, it grows on its own and can make us feel strange and crazy in all kinds of ways that we don't understand. When you start telling yourself that this feather house has to be very precise, you are basically telling yourself that unless you can make a perfect house, you will make no house at all. Once you start to think that you can't make the house perfect, you feel like your life has been defeated and that you are cursed. Then you feel like your life is over, as if you can't get up and do anything because it won't be right. All because somebody criticized that here was a little ice left on the sidewalk. That's how curses work.

TAMÁS: [Nodding] I didn't realize. I didn't know she cursed me, that she could be that mean.

BRAD: I don't think she meant to do it. It could be that when she realized she would lose her husband it also became hard for her to see you because you reminded her of him. It's possible that it became just as difficult to see you as it was to lose her husband. That's why I call it an accidental curse.

TAMÁS: At the same time, she misses me. When my younger brother visits her, she asks him why I am not around. At first, I tried to bring someone with me to help minimize the tension, because when other people were present she wasn't hurtful.

BRAD: I'm going to tell you what you need to do to break the curse and what you have to do in order to protect yourself from ever being touched by this curse again. It comes from very old Japanese wisdom. There is an old, traditional practice in Japan that when something is made, the craftsman puts a little flaw in it on purpose. If something has a little flaw while the rest of it is perfect, this is regarded as real perfection. In other words, real perfection includes a purposeful flaw. If, when you shoveled the snow, you had been Japanese you would have said to yourself, "I'm going to make sure I leave a little extra ice so that it's not perfect." Then when she saw it and criticized it you would have thought to yourself, "Ah yes, it's perfect." It would have been a confirmation that you did it perfectly, and you would have been protected from the curse. [Brad smiles]

TAMÁS: Sometimes when I build things I leave a little imperfection in it. This gives me a good feeling.

BRAD: Ah! You are Japanese! [Brad, Hillary, and Tamás laugh]

TAMÁS: It's like creating a little disorder in order to maintain the order. [Tamás takes a short pause] I'd like to tell you, that you are both very often in my mind. I see you two—you and your dear wife. You have had a very strong effect on me. My facial memory is not the best and I usually do not remember faces, but your faces are strongly in my mind, like the strongest photographs that ever existed. Since our last session I have often thought—and maybe this sounds silly and I beg your pardon—that it would be so good to live on the same street as both of you, to see you and just be able to say, "Hello." [Tamás begins to weep].

BRAD: You truly are a man who deserves a feather, a special feather. Because we have a special connection and our hearts touch each other, I'm going to ask you to break the spell. It's going to require two steps. First, you must finish the feather house as if someone's life depends on it. When you finish it, you must purposefully leave an imperfection. That should be done within one week from now. Second, you must find a nice card to send your father's wife. Maybe it has a beautiful photo of a flower or a feather on it.

HILLARY: Actually, it's best to get a card and put a feather in it. Send it to her. Not only must it be a kind card with a feather, but you must sign it, "Thinking of you," and then sign your name. Here is the important part: You must misspell your name in some small way.

TAMÁS: Shall I, for example, add an extra "m" in my name?

BRAD: Sure. You can do it however you want. This will break the spell. You have to intentionally be kind with her, share with her a feather that you find, and make an imperfection when you spell your name. And you must finish the feather house. Okay?

TAMÁS: Okay. Yes, I will do it.

BRAD: I don't know how strong this spell is, but if you find that after you do this you start to feel a little down, the second you feel that you must send her another card with another feather with your name misspelled again. And start building the house for the feather.

TAMÁS: Okay.

BRAD: Once the feather house is built, you will need another project. You need to always have a building project waiting for you because you're a man who needs to be busy with his hands.

TAMÁS: That is so right and so true. That is the hardest for me. I need to always be doing something all the time. Whenever I am not doing something, the bad thoughts come back. Whenever I have a project—even a small one—it is a good thing for me. Even mowing the lawn, for example. When I mow the lawn and then see what I have done, it gives me a good feeling.

BRAD: You know what I'm thinking? Once you build this feather house, you should build another feather house. And then another, and then another. Because I know that Hillary and I would love to have a feather house and I know others who would love to have one, too.

HILLARY: The way you describe this feather house is amazing. It could change a room. Having a feather house like that would make any room magical. You can become well-known for the feather houses you build and give to people. Take a photograph of each one, so you have a scrapbook of all the feather houses you have built. If you can make a feather house like the one you described, then you should be making more feather houses. This would be wonderful.

TAMÁS: [He nods, then is silent for a moment] Let's get back to my father's wife. What if she calls me after I send her the card and asks me, "Why did you write me after such a long time has passed? And why did you send me a feather and misspell your name?" What should I say? We have not talked for quite a long time.

BRAD: You could say, "You were the wife of my father. Every once in a while, I really miss my father. Since you were close to him, every so often I think of you." That's all you have to say.

TAMÁS: You mean I should say that I was close to my father and now that is why I think of her?

BRAD: No, you can say that now that he is gone you sometimes miss him, and this makes you think of her.

TAMÁS: What if she asks me why I don't visit his grave?

BRAD: You can say anything you wish. Anything you say is fine.

TAMÁS: But I'm afraid that she will attack me again because I am the one who broke the relationship. When she calls the house, my wife picks up the phone and I refuse to talk to her.

HILLARY: Do you hear what you are saying? What you are saying is that she has put a spell on you. The only way for you to break the spell is for you to initiate the action and always include a little imperfection. If she calls you, make sure that at least one of the things you say is not perfect.

TAMÁS: I will probably say more than one thing that is not perfect. [Tamás chuckles] I should write on the card, "I am thinking of you" and then spell my name wrong. To me, this might be interpreted as a sign that I am trying to make peace with her. [Brad begins to speak but Tamás interrupts] Sorry for interrupting, but I read somewhere that people who have a spell cast on them think about the spell all the time, and this makes the spell even stronger.

HILLARY: It's not necessarily about making peace with her; it's about breaking the spell. You are now breaking the curse and giving yourself protection. Remember that the curse was accidental.

BRAD: Yes, so it's very important what the card looks like. We don't want it to look too loving, but we don't want it to look too mean or cold. We want it to look like something she cannot possibly understand. Maybe it's a card with nothing on it but your words on the inside.

HILLARY: Your words and the feather.

TAMÁS: Maybe I hesitate because all my life I have asked others to resolve my problems instead of resolving them myself. I always felt too weak. By asking others to do it for me I did not have to take responsibility for the consequences.

BRAD: Do you hear what you are saying? When you feel that you are imperfect, you feel weak. It has always been this way.

TAMÁS: I feel I am not soft. I feel I am weak.

BRAD: When you express doubt about sending her a card and worry that she will call you, this just shows us that you are under a spell that needs to be broken. I have just one question: Is it time to break the spell?

TAMÁS: Yes.

HILLARY: There are two things you have to do. First, you have to finish the feather house this week and include the imperfection. Second, you must send this woman the imperfect card. If she calls you, give her an imperfect response.

TAMÁS: She would probably say, "I don't understand this. Explain it."

BRAD: And in response you can say anything you want. It doesn't matter.

TAMÁS: Maybe then she might say, "I don't believe you."

BRAD: If you don't know what to say then I recommend saying, "I don't know what to say, but I will explain it in the future." Very interesting. Yes? That way you don't have to know what to say. Listening to you right now, all I'm seeing and hearing is that the spell is trying to stay alive. Send her the letter and don't worry about what she says in response. Because after you send the letter, whatever she says to you will be part of the process of breaking the spell. If you don't send it, however, anything she says to you from now on under any circumstances will just make the spell stronger.

HILLARY: Your sending the letter is what sets in motion the breaking of the spell. [Tamás nods] Someday you might enjoy this so much that you are able to say to her, "Don't worry about what it means. I enjoy being crazy from time to time." [Hillary and Brad laugh] If you ever get to the point where you can easily say things like that, nobody will ever be able to put a spell on you. That's how you will sound when you are strong. You will be able to tease everybody in a good way.

TAMÁS: Yes. People would recognize that as the opposite of how I am now.

BRAD: Yes. Now I'd like you to close your eyes. I want to tell you who you are.

[Brad leans forward in his chair and grabs hold of Tamás's hand. Tamás closes his eyes. Brad speaks with more emotion and a melodic tone with a pronounced rhythm and vibration in his voice]

Deep inside, you are as soft and gentle as a feather
who can be as strong as you need to be in the right time and place.
When you were a child, you were supposed to grow up too fast.
You were expected to be too tough and too strong, too early.
But that soft child
still lives inside of you
with his feather.
When you build that home for the feather,
it will show the child inside of you
that you have built a home for him to return.
This spell was partly broken the last time we saw one another.
You felt what was possible.
Now it's time to break the spell,
to break it all the way,
and to assure that nothing can hurt you in the way it has in the past.
This means you're going to have to find many feathers for the rest of your life,
and never stop building feather houses.
Make sure they're not perfect, so you are protected.

Know that you'll touch the lives of many.
Your hands, which are strong and gentle,
will build a strong house for a gentle feather.
For this you may be known forever
as a man who lived his life like a fairy tale in Hungary.
Life is calling you to do something extraordinary,
because you understand perfection and imperfection,
and being tough and strong, as well as being soft and tender.
You understand the wind
and how things can change from a gentle breeze to a heavy storm.
You understand that now you have a very big decision—
whether you will lie down and surrender to a spell,
or whether you will spell your name incorrectly and become a living fairy tale,
an inspiration for children and parents and grandparents for all the years to come.
I can see a future, when you are buried under the ground,
after you have made all the feather houses
and become well-known for what you left behind.
I see people every week coming to your grave and placing a feather,
one by one
making a soft, feather bed.
Every once in a while those feathers blow into the hills
across the rivers
carried by the wind whether gentle or strong
falling into the hands of little boys whose fathers are too strict,
taking the feather home,
finding themselves carried through because they, too, know that's how your story began. So, we bless your life.
We ask that you take a stand for everyone's life that you can touch,
because of everything that has happened to you,
and who you really are.
[There is a long silence while Tamás slowly opens his eyes. Brad releases his hand. Tamás wipes tears from his eyes and takes a deep breath]

TAMÁS: Thank you, thank you so much.

Brad, Hillary, and Tamás stand and embrace.

One week later, Tamás brought the house he built for the feather to show us, and we took this photograph:

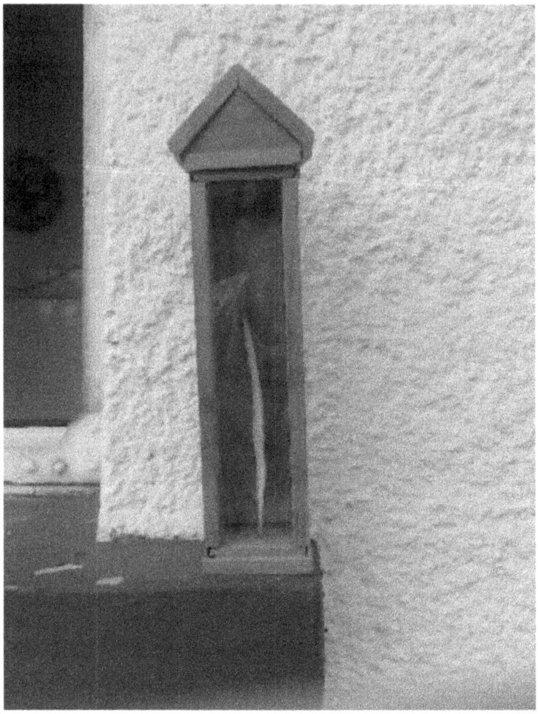

We invite you to incorporate this teaching about softness into your creative therapy future. Find your own feather and then either build a feather house or find a large enough piece of paper to sketch the outline of one so that your feather fits inside its drawn walls. Place this feather and its dwelling place in a safe place. If this seems too childish a task for you, then go have a piece of sour cherry pie in order to activate your childlike wonder and eagerness to take on this magical project. Find the feather and make it a home—not only for yourself, but for someone whose life may be transformed by the gentle surprise it is capable of delivering. Wonder about what client or struggling therapist you will meet in the future with whom you can share the feather story and reveal your feather home. See this as hosting more than a feather—here also resides the feather teaching of Tamás.

Make sure that what you build or draw, as well as the story you tell, has an imperfection. This will help break the spell or curse that any adult part of your mind might have put on your successful completion of this creative mission. Also know that whenever you are too hard on yourself with criticism, doubt, or lack of inspiration, use your feather to tickle you. You might have to ask someone to tickle you with it and help make you soft again. As one tickle leads to the next tickle, one feather brings forth more feathers found by other people, including you. As feathers are gathered and housed throughout the world, we may someday find that no one ever feels alone for "birds of a feather flock together." Perhaps more importantly, as Emily Dickinson said, "Hope is the thing with feathers; that perches in the soul." Why bother with a feather? When asked why she became a writer, Rene Char answered both questions, "A bird's feather on my windowpane in winter and all at once there arose in my heart a battle of embers never to subside again." You must soften and make your heart ready to be touched by both a musical note and a feather flight. Let a feather lead the way to bringing this change home. If you build it, creative wisdom will come.

8

THE INTESTINAL FRIEND

A young woman from Budapest came to us seeking help with her anxiety and chronic diarrhea, considered a psychosomatic intestinal disorder that made it difficult for her to stay in a social situation for very long. The psychiatrist who had been working with her made the referral. When we met she apologized in advance, saying she might have to excuse herself several times during the session to run to the bathroom.

BRAD: Thank you for coming.

HILLARY: Please, let us know what you'd like to talk about today.

NORA: I have been struggling with anxiety. I get really anxious, and it gives me diarrhea. I can't live the way I'd like to. I can't even stay long in a room.

BRAD: Excuse me, can I just ask for clarification—does your anxiety cause diarrhea? Or does your diarrhea make you anxious?

NORA: I don't really know anymore. I think sometimes the anxiety causes it, but sometimes I think it's the other way around.

HILLARY: Of course, that's the way it is.

NORA: I take medication for it now.

HILLARY: Medication for the diarrhea or for the anxiety?

NORA: It's for the anxiety and sometimes it's for the diarrhea. Basically, I feel like I don't have a life anymore and I don't know how to change it.

BRAD: So, what if you could stop the diarrhea, but you would still be anxious?

HILLARY: Or what if you could stop the anxiety, but still have the diarrhea—which would you prefer? We're just curious.

NORA: Okay. [Nora thinks for a second] Stop the diarrhea.

BRAD: Well it's very interesting that we see you this morning, because I woke up in the middle of the night thinking what I want to say to you today. It's always a good sign when the recommendation comes from a mysterious intuition arriving in the middle of the night. I haven't even shared this with Hillary because I want it to be said for the first time with you present so it feels fresh and alive. This is what I woke up imagining I'd say to you: Many years ago, I became friends with a very famous medical doctor in the United States. He is no longer alive, but he was one of the most famous medical doctors in the world. He had his own large clinic in Palm Beach where he worked with every kind of patient. Some were dying while other patients had unusual symptoms. Every imaginable issue was treated at that clinic. His name was Dr. John Upledger. He had medical research grants funded by the government and other medical foundations. About twenty or thirty years ago when "holistic," "complementary," or "integrative" medicine became popular, the government chose a small group of prestigious doctors to oversee research in this area and he was one of them. One year the chairman of Dr. Upledger's board decided that she would gift him some time with me for his birthday present. So, they paid me to come spend one week with him. One of the reasons for this was that he loved jazz piano, especially Erroll Garner, and he was interested in healing. They had discovered I also had these interests, so they flew me out. We were first introduced at a mansion on beachfront property near Miami. There was a grand piano there, so we took turns playing the piano for each other. Then we talked. We got to know each other quite well. He had made several important medical discoveries in his work with children, adults, and the elderly. He worked with cancer, asthma, spinal conditions, bowel conditions, mental conditions—he worked with everything. At the end of our week together he said he would now share his biggest discovery. What he said is what I woke up hearing in the middle of the night, thinking I should tell you today. He told me he had found a special means of working with the body. His words were this: "The patient should have a conversation with the organ or part of the body that is causing them trouble." I was surprised and replied, "What?" Dr. Upledger answered, "I'm totally serious. If you are having a problem with an organ you should talk to it—talk to the whole organ." I said, "Well, John, what should the patient say to the organ?" He replied, "It should be personal, it should be respectful, and it should express gratitude. What you say should show that you appreciate that the organ knows something that you don't know. This keeps you from getting too bossy and making it irritated about your being uppity. For example, you don't want to say to your stomach, "Stomach, stop that ache. I hate it!" That will not please the stomach who is only trying to help. The stomach knows that it gave you that ache in order to help you, in order to draw your attention to something that needs to be done differently. If you don't pay attention, the stomach will just keep sending the ache. So first say, "Stomach, I know you're trying to help me, and I thank you for all of your help." [Nora laughs and continues smiling] "But I think there is a possibility that maybe you have done your job, so you don't have to feel like you need to keep making the ache. The ache doesn't need to stay around any longer because I got the message. Thank you." [Nora laughs again] Dr. Upledger told me that it's very important how you talk to your body because if you don't express enough appreciation and gratitude, the organ will feel like you don't yet understand or have not received the help the symptom meant to offer. And if you exaggerate the way you talk, it will just think, "Oh, you're just teasing me. You don't really mean it, you're just pretending." So it's very important that you have a heart to heart, respectful, appreciative conversation with your organ. This was the important secret this famous medical doctor shared with me and we are passing on to you. If I told you this in the beginning without telling you more about this doctor, you would have thought it was crazy advice. But I can tell you that Dr. Upledger was very famous and he helped a lot of people. People with cancer of the liver, for example, would speak to their liver in a personal, heartfelt way. In your case, you would be talking to your intestines. Is that right?

NORA: Yes, that's right.

HILLARY: You would have a personal conversation with your intestine. To make it personal, you can choose a name for your intestines that sounds more engaging.

NORA: [Smiling, lights up] Oh!

BRAD: We'll let you think about that for a minute. You can choose a name that feels more personal and intimate for both you and your intestines.

HILLARY: You don't just want to say, "Hey, intestines let's talk." [Nora laughs] That doesn't sound or feel like a real personal conversation. That would sound weird.

BRAD: First, I'd like to ask you, would it be the name of a man or of a woman? [There is a silent pause as Nora thinks about it]

HILLARY: What do you think feels more true? A man's name or a woman's name?
NORA: A man's name.
HILLARY: Would it be a boy, a young man, or an old man?
NORA: Someone young.
BRAD: Someone young—how young?
NORA: Someone my age. [Nora is in her late twenties]
BRAD: Would it be a local name? Or foreign?
NORA: [Answers immediately]. Hungarian.
BRAD: So it would be a young man, your age, who is Hungarian.
NORA: Yes.
HILLARY: Would it be someone who lives in the area where you live, or in a different part of the country?
NORA: My area.
BRAD: Okay. Would it be someone who is muscular—
HILLARY: Perhaps good looking?
NORA: [Smiles and then laughs] Yes. Why not?
[At this point, Nora does not pause to think, but answers quickly]
BRAD: And what about his hair color?
NORA: Brown.
HILLARY: Would it be short or long?
NORA: Short.
BRAD: Very good. And if this young man had gone to college, what subject would you guess that he studied? Let me ask you—is he a college graduate?
NORA: Yes.
BRAD: Okay, what subject did he study?
NORA: Architecture.
HILLARY: And what is his favorite music?
NORA: Probably pop music from the 80s and 90s.
HILLARY: Does he enjoy poetry?
NORA: No.
HILLARY: Does he like to dance?
NORA: No.
HILLARY: How about sports? Does he like sports?
NORA: Yes.
BRAD: Which one?
NORA: Any kind.
BRAD: Would he rather throw a ball or kick a ball.
NORA: Throw a ball.
HILLARY: Okay. Is he tall or short?
NORA: Tall.
HILLARY: Very tall, or just a little tall?

NORA: Just a little tall—taller than I am.

BRAD: Very good. And if you had to guess his favorite book, what would it be?

NORA: I'm not sure.

BRAD: If you had to guess—let's just say you had to go to a bookstore and buy him a book that you hoped he would say, "This is the best book I have ever read," what would you guess? Would it be a funny book or a serious book?

NORA: A serious book.

BRAD: About history or contemporary things?

NORA: Not history.

BRAD: So something modern, maybe from the 80s?
[Nora and everyone laugh]

NORA: I'm not sure, I can't choose.

HILLARY: This is very good, because you have just created someone you can personally relate to. Now give him his name. What name do you choose for this man?

NORA: [Answers immediately] Janos.

BRAD: Janos?

NORA: Yes.

BRAD: So are you ready to be someone who tries this experiment?

NORA: Yes, yes.

BRAD: By now, we should all agree that you have probably tried everything else there is to try for your condition. There probably are no more medical tests left, and no more medications left. It's time for you to try this famous doctor's last secret. Dr. Upledger is no longer living and this was the last secret about medicine he offered us. You are to solemnly pledge to not call this organ an intestine. Forever, for the rest of your life, you should never ever call it your intestine. Never again shall this name be spoken. If you ever catch yourself thinking or talking to someone about your intestine or gut, then immediately stop. Stop this very second.

HILLARY: You need to always use the name, Janos—the name of that man, who is about your age, who is taller than you, who majored in architecture, who likes all sports, who prefers to throw the ball rather than kick it, who enjoys the music of the 80s and 90s, who would prefer a contemporary rather than historical book. Who is someone you have just gotten to know. This is someone you need to have a conversation with. And this conversation must start by calling his name, saying, "Hello, Janos."

BRAD: You need to say something like, "I know that you came to me and you made me notice that something is going on down here.

I appreciate that you came to help me. I'm sorry I tried to push you away and not pay attention, and the more I did that the more you said, "I'm here, I'm just trying to help." You could also say, "I think, Janos, that you have helped me. And I just want you to know that I appreciate that, so I say thank you."

NORA: And what if I don't feel this way?

BRAD: You must if you want to follow the doctor's final advice. This part of you needs to hear that the rest of you can acknowledge that its action isn't random or dumb; it has a reason. Though you may never fully understand any of this, you can choose to follow the good doctor's advice and express your appreciation for what that organ is trying to do—it's trying to get an important message through. Again, recognize that the communication of Janos is there for a reason, so show your appreciation even though you may never understand it.

HILLARY: You can apologize for not having talked to it earlier. You must say in some way—and this is the important part—"I think you have done your job. You can go on and help somebody else now." [Nora laughs] This is very important.

BRAD: Because what this doctor discovered was that the human body is not stupid. There is wisdom in the human body and there is wisdom in every uncomfortable and comfortable experience it offers. He knew that whatever created you, whatever universe or whatever creator made you, was not stupid. Medical science also now knows that every disease is partly a medicine that helps the body make a correction or adjustment. They don't know why sometimes it sticks around so long. Even after the adjustment is made, it may still hang around. You might wonder, "What is that cold or flu doing?" Some scientists say that it is exercising your ability to self-heal. But it doesn't matter if you understand or know. All you need to know is that the body is not stupid.

HILLARY: And what this doctor figured out is that it's smart to talk to it with utmost sincerity and say, "Thank you! I know you came for a reason, which I can't understand, but I feel now that your job is done, you can go help someone else, and I appreciate what you have done."

BRAD: And—now this is going to be even harder to do—you have to also say, "If you need a little more time, I understand. But just know that I'm paying attention to you, now." Strange things happen to people when they do this. Sometimes they have a dream where that person they spoke to comes to them in a dream and says, "I've just been trying to help you learn how to let go of things you don't need." Or, "I've been trying to distract you from

something that's taking too much of your attention." It could be any message. It might speak in a language you don't understand, like [Brad speaks gibberish] "Maka, ju ju gee." It might speak in sign language or smoke signals or foghorns or volcanic eruptions or fire alarms or traffic lights or anything at all. Then you wake up and realize that you had a dream, thinking, "I feel funny, I feel different." You might even feel weird if you had a whole month or week where you had no diarrhea—you might start missing Janos. This is a weird thing that sometimes happens to people. They can get so close to their sickness that they actually miss it when it leaves. Some people miss prison when they are let out. You might miss Janos if he stops communicating.
[Nora is nodding, smiling slightly]

HILLARY: I think a deep part of you already knows about who's inside of you. Because when we asked you to describe Janos, you knew many things about him—he's a young, tall, architect who loves sports and music and lives in Budapest. This is a man that many women your age in Budapest would like to meet and hang out with. I think if you put an ad in the newspaper with a description of Janos and an invitation to meet him, you would have a line of young women outside the door. [Nora and everyone laugh] The way you described Janos made me think that when you have that conversation with him, you would want to light some candles and maybe even buy some roses. I know you and Janos are still working out your relationship, and that you're still figuring out how much longer you'd like Janos to be around, but I think that, based on the way you were able to describe him, and how well you know him, that some part of you does feel an appreciation for what he has brought to your life. [Nora giggles and nods]

BRAD: I just had a funny thought. [Turning to Hillary] Now I wouldn't recommend she actually do this, but I can imagine a short story about a woman just like her having this same identical conversation. Imagine that after the session she actually did go to a dating service and gave this exact description, this time depicting the man she wants to date herself. Then bam—up comes this photograph of a man fitting the description. The dating service then surprisingly says, "Here's your intestine." [Everyone erupts in laughter] That would be very crazy.

HILLARY: We can't say such a thing should happen or would happen but thinking about it does open up all kinds of possibilities. But you know what? Dr. Upledger prescribed this treatment for a lot of people and their condition changed. And you know what? He wrote a book on it, about talking to your cells. I don't know if you're ready for Janos to come out of hiding, or whether you're fine living in the dark. I'm not sure if you're ready to have the conversation. Are you?

NORA: Right now?

HILLARY: Yes, why not?

BRAD: Are you ready? [Nora is silent] Maybe it's too early? Maybe you would like another week. In all seriousness, what if you had this conversation and everything you have been worried about left. Your diarrhea left, your anxiety left, all the things you get anxious about left. All of it just left. It might be too big of a shock to you, for it to happen so quickly. I don't know, I'm just asking. There are therapists who ask that question.

NORA: I understand.

HILLARY: So I guess the first question is, are you ready to introduce yourself to Janos?

NORA: Yes.

BRAD: That's a start.

[Nora nods, takes a deep breath, closes her eyes, and begins talking to Janos]

NORA: Janos, we have known each other for a long time. You came in to my life when I was going through some stress at work and in my personal life. And I know you have tried to show me the things I need to learn. I have tried to learn what you have wanted to teach me. I have also tried everything to make you go away, but I could not. I failed every time. So, I would like to say that I recognize that maybe there is something more that you have to teach me. As funny as it is to say, I have evolved because of you. I'm more patient, I understand people better, and I have more empathy. In some way I am actually calmer, even though inside I feel anxious. I think have already learned enough and I would just like to go on with my life without you … if that is okay with you.

BRAD: That's right.

HILLARY: Good. It's so important you said that it's okay for you if he has to stay a bit longer, but also that it's okay with you if he goes.

BRAD: I'd like you to keep your eyes closed. [Brad leans forward and takes hold of Nora's hand. He switches tone and speaks as he moves her hand to help induce a kinetic trance] Now we invite you to imagine that Janos answers back and says, "I came to help you the best way I know how. To distract you from that which held you back. To remind you that there is more of you than is seen or heard. To try to catch your attention to show you that there is more you can do and more you can learn, which I'm so happy to hear has taken place. But know—I have grown anxious about you. Sometimes it's hard for me to leave you for fear that you'll be anxious without me. In other words, I'm having a hard time letting go. But if I truly can be told, and if I truly hear, and if I truly feel, and if I truly see that you are no longer in need of me, then I must go, as sad as that would be for me … But I'm so happy today that you know I'm not a weak sickness, but that I'm a strong man. I'm so glad today that you know that I have been here to help you and that you have been able to acknowledge that some of that help has made your life not only different, but also better. It's so good to know that you spoke tenderly to me, sweetly to me, and I want you to know that I don't have to leave and never see you again, because there may be a time in your life that you need me to help. You just might find yourself in an impossible situation someday where you don't have the courage to just get up and leave the room. If that happens, you can call on my name and I'll be right there and give you a reason to leave. But there is no need when you feel that you have received all that I can teach and all that I have to offer.

… Now I'm listening to this different way you are now speaking to me. I am so relieved that you no longer fear me or despise me or curse me. You know that I was only doing my job, which is to help. So, if you don't mind, maybe in the next week or two or three, but especially now, if you don't mind, in order to help me feel this is real, I need to hear more from you. Especially when you're alone, because then I'll know you are doing this because you chose to, not just because people who are trying to help you are suggesting you talk to me. I really need to know that you chose to do it yourself, so tonight and tomorrow morning and the next afternoon, I really want to hear you say my name. I want to hear you play me a song from the 80s. I want to hear you and see you turn on the television and find a sport that I'd like to watch for a few minutes. I want you to write me a letter. I want you to sing to me. I want you to hum to me. I want to hear the sincerity of the whole of you, so I can be assured, and myself no longer feel anxious about you. Hopefully you'll believe that I can always return whenever you need me if you call on my name. But I'll only come if you call my name. That's the way the cells of the body, the organs of the body, the mystery of the body, works in relationship to the whole of you and the whole of life. So, it's up to you for I will be waiting each morning, day, and night, to hear and see and feel something from you. You can even go to the bakery and choose something sweet for me to eat. You can even surprise me with something that I never would expect.

But please, forever more, call me by my true name, and know that I came to ease not bring disease, though the challenge of learning is never easy.

[Brad releases Nora's hand. She slowly opens her eyes]

BRAD: That's a strange thing to wake up in the middle of the night and remember, isn't it?

NORA: Yes.

HILLARY: Maybe one of the ways Janos will know that you are okay, and you are ready for Janos to move on when it's time, is that he sees that you have found a different way of being in relationship to the different parts of you. Someday, for example, you might find you have to have another conversation with another part of you that has brought you a different lesson. You're entering a whole new world, a whole new way of being in relationship to every part of you. But for now, you don't need to think about that. You only need to have some conversations with Janos.

BRAD: Hillary is right, because if you learn to talk in this kind of deep way to deeper parts of you, you'll be teaching yourself how to have deeper conversations when those opportunities arrive and are needed. The way you talk to Janos now will teach you even more lessons for the future of your life. Are you a writer?

NORA: No, why?

BRAD: Because you have the mind for description, like a writer.

HILLARY: Maybe you should write down all the descriptions you made of Janos today as if you were making a detailed description for a detective.

BRAD: Wouldn't that be something, if you could write a five-page description and hire a detective to find this person? [Brad and Nora laugh]

HILLARY: That would be very, very interesting. That would be an interesting story for a movie. It's strange how things happen to our bodies and to our minds and hearts that are beyond our understanding and outside our consciousness—deep knowing, deep communication, and deep relationships within. When we strive to be the best person we can become, sometimes we notice there are certain things about us that there should be less of. You mentioned in your thanks to Janos that you have become more patient and less impatient. You might want to tell your doctor the next time you see him that you are no longer the same because there is more of you alive—you are now his patience.

NORA: Yes!

BRAD: It's not all that surprising to hear that this special character came into your life during a time when you had certain things you wanted to let go of and certain things you wanted less of. This character showed up to help you let go of all that needed to go as it also searched to help you find more inside and outside of you …

HILARY: We really think that you should do all these things—flood your week with conversations, talks, walks, songs, and other special encounters and creative interactions with Janos. It's time for you to be in charge of this relationship. Janos has been shouting at you to get your attention and you have been looking in the other direction. This made him pursue you that much more.

NORA: [Nodding and smiling] Yes, yes.

BRAD: That's an old courtship game. [Everyone laughs]Now it's time for you to be the one in charge. You do the talking. He'll be in shock, but you're going to have a different relationship. Because now when he tries to get your attention, you'll answer back and put him in his right place, but you'll answer with sweetness and with appreciation, and with wisdom, also giving him the permission to go help someone else. That's what an old medical doctor, who was also a famous healer, would suggest to you if he were in this room right now.

NORA: Thank you. Thank you.

BRAD: I actually tried this myself once and it worked. Then I doubted it and my problem came back, so I had to do it again. [Brad laughs] You can communicate with your body but be sincere and make sure you endear rather than endure it.

HILLARY: Most of us are just walking heads and we think that everything is just on top. We only talk to our brains. But the rest of our body is trying to say, "Hey! I'm here down below! I'm here too!" There is more to you than just this [points to head] but we look at the body like it's some mystery that we shouldn't be polite to or respect. We only yell at it or go to war with it. "Stop it! Would you stop bothering me!" We never say, "Hello. Thank you for all you are trying to teach me, and all that you are trying to remind me of that is important that I too often forget."

BRAD: Thank you for bringing us a reminder of the body we may never understand. But we must remember that the body is not stupid, nor is the universe that made it. What is the size of the intestine? How many meters long?

DEZSOE: The whole intestine?

BRAD: [Whispers] Oops—I'm not supposed to say that word.

DEZSOE: About 12 meters.

BRAD: Wow, Janos is a tall man! [Everyone laughs] He is a giant!

HILLARY: A tall, good looking athlete. I think you should also go find at least three jokes that Janos will enjoy.

BRAD: Yes. When Janos is asleep, go on the internet and find some good jokes. You'll know what kind of joke is the right kind for him. Then write them down and read it out loud to him. Because if he sees you teasing him, he'll know you're better. The more you worry about all this, the more anxious you get about all this, the more anxious and worried Janos will be for you, and the longer he'll stick around. Do you see the trap?

NORA: Yes.

BRAD: Go tell Janos some jokes, hopefully jokes about a very tall man. [Everyone laughs]

HILLARY: And some architect jokes, if there is such a thing. [Everyone laughs]

BRAD: And sports jokes.

HILLARY: And jokes that have a surprise ending.

BRAD: It's time for you to begin.
[Hillary and Brad stand up and embrace Nora]

NORA: Thank you, yes.

It's time for you to have a conversation with whatever parts of your body have become unconscious and have likely grown tired of trying to get your attention to receive whatever they wish you'd offer a session. Stop listening only to your gut and your head, and start listening to your palms, fingertips, arms, and the soles of your feet, to mention a few neglected body parts. The Kalahari Bushmen call these body communications "tappings." They, likely more than anyone else, find the body's conversations as more meaningful than the chitchat going on above. A Bushman hunter will feel a tapping on an arm that signals it is time to hunt. At other times it is felt as an itch in the palm when someone is on the way with a gift or a tingle in the calves when it is time for a healing dance. Our fieldwork actually studied the body dictionary of the Bushmen (B. Keeney & H. Keeney, 2015).

The creative therapist also learns to experience the creative tappings that knock on the body throughout a session. You feel fidgety when your body wants more action. At other times you feel sleepy when you are ready to drop a therapy model and paddle through an improvisational current. When your calves remind you they are present, take a stand and get out of that chair. Or if a finger twitches, randomly point to anything. If your back suddenly aches, turn around and face a new front. If your head aches, stop interpreting. Whenever words seem stuck, don't speak. Draw a sketch instead. Need to take a stretch? Why resist when it might extend the room? If thirsty for a glass of water, jump into the creative sea. If feeling the slow burden of getting through the hour, then pass the verbiage and ask the client to change. Have them at least walk around the room or randomly pull a book off the shelf and open it to any page so only its unexpected sentence steers the next things said. In other words, why always say it when your body can better play with it?

Go all the way and make the whole of your body your co-therapist. Give it a name. If not Janos, then how about adopting a ghost from the past? We often ask trainees what ancestor from the past, from saint to master healer, they would choose to sit by their side in a session. Who would you choose? The Buddha or Emily Dickenson? Miles Davis for extending the range or Buddy Rich to rhythmically enrich? Do you want more than one or two helpers? Go ahead and build an all-star ghost team. These ghosts are excellent hosts and are ready to step into your space and be an unconscious influence on how you can more creatively change. Put their portraits on the wall as a reminder of who is there with you. Embody creative action by performing it, but this time not alone. Hear creatively, see creatively, and feel creatively by sincerely acting like its real.

If you can't stop interpreting, then consider it verbal diarrhea. Talk to your intestine about it. But before you do so, rename it. Perhaps call it Agent 007 (or if you must, call it Agent 002) and presume it works for another kind of intelligence agency. It might advise you to find a wider panorama that enables more of the whole creative landscape to be experienced. Or create a diorama where three-dimensional characters arrive. If you want the meat of action, leave the word salad behind. Better yet, serve that word salad and only let go of its meaning. Before there is room to create, all the theoretical sneaky poo needs to be let go. Thank your intestinal cybernetic loop for its important recycling of truth. In all seriousness, it's time to get more of your organs involved in a session. This is especially true for your heart and even more so for your soul. Clear the deck, open the sail, and have a date with the rest of you!

9

SHARING THE BITTERNESS UNTIL DEATH DO US PART

Ádám and Ilona are a young Hungarian couple in their late twenties living in Budapest. They were engaged to be married one month from the date of this session, which was conducted in front of an audience in Budapest.

BRAD: So, who would like to speak first?

[Ádám and Ilona look at each other and laugh. Ilona points to Ádám]

ÁDÁM: Okay, I guess I'll volunteer. Well, we have heard a lot about you both, and we've been looking forward to meeting you.

BRAD: It's nice to meet you both.

ÁDÁM: Thank you. Our wedding will be the beginning of August, about one month from now.

HILLARY: Congratulations!

ÁDÁM AND ILONA: [In unison] Thank you.

ÁDÁM: We have known Dezsoe for a long time and he has helped both of us a lot, together and separately. [Dezsoe Birkas, our colleague, is present in the audience]

ILONA: [pointing to Ádám] He was the first person to see Dezsoe.

ÁDÁM: Yes. Ten years ago, I came to see Dezsoe twice because I got panic attacks for no reason; they came out of thin air. I had gone to many other doctors and they thought I had all kinds of problems, maybe even a brain tumor. I saw Dezsoe twice and he helped me so much that the panic attacks stopped. He gave me some exercises to do that I thought were crazy, but doing them is what healed me. Then I stopped coming to see him. Two years later, Dezsoe called me out of the blue, and it felt really good to reconnect with him, so I began seeing him again. A very strong bond developed between us. I learned to deal with the panic attacks and I don't have them anymore. I am a lawyer, and my fiancée and I are fine, it's just that the feeling of freedom, pleasure, and joy is somehow missing from my life and from our lives together. Four years ago, Ilona and I met, and we were really different. But even so, we grew closer and closer. We also have had many fights. I have always lived my life in a way where I don't really say what I am feeling or what I really need. I have always tried to be sensitive and accept everybody else's wishes and needs, but now it has become a problem. Now there are problems between us as a couple.

ILONA: I always tell him that this is a problem—that he doesn't say what he is feeling or what he needs. Finally, it is good to hear him say that he knows this is a problem! [Ilona and Ádám both laugh]

BRAD: [Interrupting the laughter, Brad holds up his hand] Just a minute. One of the things I want to share before I forget it is that when you [speaking to Ádám] said "panic attack," my mind heard, "panic visit." You have had panic visits. Then I wondered what is it about you that is able to successfully invite so many things. Perhaps every experience in the world wants to come visit you? Are you such a nice guy that you have a sign hanging around your neck that says, "Everyone Welcome" so that even panic makes a visit? [Ilona and Ádám laugh] This is what went through my mind. I don't know what this means, I just wanted to share with you that this is what went through my mind. It's interesting that you can make so many experiences and people want to come visit, including Mr. Panic. [Speaking to Ilona] Is this true about him?

ILONA: Yes, of course. When I saw him for the first time I saw that he had a force, a power, an energy or life energy. I was in a very difficult time in my life and I wanted that energy. I wanted to be part of his life and to be so full of energy and happiness. He was always laughing and in a good mood.

ÁDÁM: During the last four years, our relationship has been up and down, but we have been more up than down. We would laugh a lot, then argue, and then be laughing again. I think what we need is to get more calm.

ILONA: Yes, we need to find a balance.

ÁDÁM: Yes.

ILONA: We are either very up or very down.

ÁDÁM: I think the main problem is that she is nervous, and I don't know how to help her. When she is nervous, I then also feel nervous.

HILLARY: So, she has a power too.
ÁDÁM: Yes, she does. [Ádám and Ilona both laugh]
HILLARY: [Speaking to Ádám] Does your sign that says "Welcome" bring everything to you?
ÁDÁM: Yes. Good things and also bad things.
BRAD: Does your sign say, "Open 24 Hours for Everything and Anyone." [Ilona and Ádám both laugh]
ÁDÁM: Yes, and that's one of the biggest issues that I have been working on in therapy—learning how to say no to people. It's hard for me because I don't want to be a bad guy. I want to be the good guy who is always friendly.
BRAD: [Speaking to Ilona] Maybe you need to make another sign for him that says, "Closed. Open tomorrow at 9 a.m." [The couple and the audience laugh] I'm serious. Because he doesn't know when the shop needs to be open or closed.
ÁDÁM: That's why I cannot go home on time at night. I feel I should stay out more and more. I don't want to hurt Ilona, but she thinks that I am hurting her when I don't come home.
HILLARY: Do you mean that you are working late?
ILONA: No, he means he doesn't want to come home from the club hanging out with friends! [Ilona and Ádám both laugh]
BRAD: [Speaking to Ádám] Well, this is the trap you're in. You are tricking yourself. You don't see that the more open you are, the more closed you actually are. Because when you are open for one thing, you are closed for another. If you're open to being awake, you're closed to being asleep. When you are open to play, you are closed to work. [Brad turns to Ilona] I'm going to tell you something about Ádám that he probably doesn't know about himself: He is a very closed person. He is closed because he is so open in other areas of his life. It's a strange thing, yes? He is so open that craziness of all kinds can show up, like panic, or waking up in the middle of the night worrying whether he is doing the right thing. [Speaking now to Ádám] Does worry wake you up in the night?
ÁDÁM: Yes.
BRAD: [Brad nods and then speaks to Ilona] So when he comes home is he still out? Or does all of him come home?
ILONA: None of him comes home. All of him is with his friends partying at night.
HILLARY: So, the bar is open all night?
ILONA: Yes, and then I am very furious and very angry with him about coming home so late. I am wondering why he has to be out with friends so late? Of course, I know that it doesn't help if I get angry, because that doesn't make him come home earlier. I think

he is out with friends knowing that I'm waiting for him at home angry, so he stays out even later. I know I don't need to behave like this, but I can't control my anger.

HILLARY: [Speaking to Ilona] Do you sometimes start to feel panic?

ILONA: Yes, I started to feel panic. For example, I never used to be afraid of flying, but now when I fly I get panic attacks.

BRAD: [Speaking to Ádám] Did you know that she was feeling panic?

ÁDÁM: She told me about it once, I think.

BRAD: [Speaking to Ilona] How many times have you experienced it?

ILONA: Two or three times. It's a very bad feeling. Ádám told me before how bad it feels, but until I experienced it I didn't know.

ÁDÁM: I feel badly about it because I don't have panic anymore.

HILLARY: That's because she has it now.

[Ilona and Ádám both laugh]

BRAD: [Speaking to Ilona] Maybe you should give it back to him.

[The couple laughs again]

HILLARY: [Speaking to Ilona] Would you know what to do to make him panic?

ILONA: Yes—to fight a lot with him and make him nervous, or to make him feel that our life together is not good and that we are arguing too much and don't have a good balance. That would make him panic.

BRAD: You know what I think the fight is really about? It's about who owns the panic. [Ilona and Ádám both laugh] You both argue back and forth as if saying, "You take the panic," "No *you* take the panic." Maybe instead you should share it. If both of you had half the panic things would be different. Really. [Ilona nods, and then Brad speaks directly to her] In addition to a sign for Ádám to wear that says, "open" and "closed," my fantasy is that you buy Ádám a new watch. Instead of the time, it just tells him when he's open and when he's closed. [Ilona and Ádám laugh] Because if he is closed when he should be open, and he's open when he should be closed, then panic knocks on your door. My fantasy is that we could take an empty bottle—one for each of you—and pour the panic so that each bottle holds half. [Speaking now to Ádám] If it were possible, would you take half of her panic?

ÁDÁM: I would take more than half.

BRAD: That would make her panic. [Brad smiles and the couple and audience laugh] If panic were a liquid, what liquid would it be? Would it be water, grape juice, lemon juice? What would it be?

ILONA: It would be Kofola. [Ádám, Ilona, and some members of the audience laugh] Kofola is kind of like Coke. Coca-Cola is good, but Kofola is awful. It's made in the Czech Republic and Slovakia.

HILLARY: Do you know where to find it?

ILONA: We would have to travel far, but yes, we could find it.

HILLARY: Then this is a trip that you need to take together. Go buy some Kofola.

BRAD: It may be the most important trip of your life.

ÁDÁM AND ILONA: [In unison] Okay.

HILLARY: I assume it's possible to do this.

ILONA: Yes.

BRAD: In addition, you should each buy two new glasses, or mugs, or steins. They should look very bad, even frightening. They should be so ugly that you think to yourself, "I don't want that glass in my house. I would never want to buy it or drink out of it." When you find these glasses or mugs, then fill each half full of this terrible tasting drink.

HILLARY: When you do this, you will then be sharing the Kofola, the bitterness of life. You will also be helping each other learn to keep the right hours. [Speaking to Ádám] Just like Ilona is going to help you know when it is time for you to be open and when it is time to be closed, you will learn that your marriage also has to keep the right hours.

BRAD: That's the most important "Open/Closed" sign to make.

HILLARY: [Ádám is nodding] Yes. Because getting married is like setting up a new shop. You both have to decide together what hours you will keep. Sometimes as a couple you are closed to the rest of the world, and sometimes you are open.

BRAD: Exactly. So, number one—most importantly—you must take a journey together to buy the scary, ugly glasses. What do you think they will be—a glass, a cup, or a stein? What do you think?

ILONA: Glass.

ÁDÁM: Cup.

[Ilona and Ádám both respond in unison, each saying the opposite. They and the audience erupt in laughter]

BRAD: Very good.

ILONA: I will have the glass and he will have the cup.

BRAD: You should go together to shop for these. You, Ilona, should try to find a cup for Ádám that he will definitely *not* like. When you think you have found it you should ask him, "Do you like this?" If he says, "No," then you should definitely buy it. You, Ádám, should find what you think Ilona won't like. This may take a long time. If you find something and hold it up to her and Ilona says, "I don't like that," then you know you should buy it. After you buy the cup and the glass, go get some of this panic drink. Maybe you have to add something to it to make it taste even worse, such as garlic.

ÁDÁM: I like garlic.

ILONA: [Making a face of disgust] I don't.

[They both laugh]

BRAD: Good, then she gets the garlic and Ilona you put something in Ádám's drink that he doesn't like. When you come home from this trip, the first thing you have to do is to put half the panic drink in the glass and half in the cup. While holding them up as if making a toast, Ádám you will say to Ilona: "I, your future husband, promise to own half the panic." He will want to say that he will own more, but Ilona you must shake your head no and only let him own half. Then, Ilona, you will say: "I, your future wife, promise to own half the panic." No less, no more. And then you each have to drink the liquid. Then fill the cup and the glass half full again and put them both in the fridge. Whenever you feel an argument come on, or you feel that Ádám is not keeping the hours, or Ádám if you feel that Ilona is not keeping the hours, this means you're both not sharing the panic. You will then both have to get out the cup and glass and go through the ritual again. I think you both understand. [Ilona and Ádám both nod] Now you have to decide, together, when this new shop will be open for business, and what hours you will keep. Do either one of you know how to draw?

ILONA: I draw sometimes, yes.

HILLARY: Perfect. Then make a little open/closed sign with hours on it that looks like a shop sign. Make two so each of you can carry it with you every day. During the day, you can each look at it to remind you when this shop [pointing to both of them] is open, and when it is closed.

ILONA: So I have to make two signs—one for each of us.

BRAD: Yes. Let's have the two of you hold hands right now. [Ilona and Ádám each grab the other's hand, and Brad then leans forward and holds their clasped hands in his. Brad speaks with a vibration in his voice. As he begins speaking, both Ilona and Ádám close their eyes] We all see the love inside both of you. We have heard that each of you has a power and a magnetism that draws the other to you. Each of you, in some unexplainable way, can even transfer your feelings from one to the other. Because you are beginning to create a new shop together, a new house, a new place, and a new life, it's very important that you always share the panic. One half for you and one half for you. No more, no less. It's good for everyone to have a little panic. The panic is a reminder when it's time for some things to open, and some things to close. It's a reminder that it's time for some things to continue, and some things to stop. It's a reminder that certain things need to wake up, and certain things need to go to sleep. It's like the school bell that rings, telling you "school is starting now," or that it's time to go home. Each of you is about to do something never done by any couple before in history. You will soon take a journey to look for an unusual cup and glass, one that each of you doesn't like. You will fill it half full of that which you don't want to drink, so you can equally share all the things in life that aren't sweet. Because that is half of life—half of life is bitter, and half of life is sweet. Some days we feel healthy, some days we are sick. Some days we are relaxed, some days we are tense. But when you share everything with one another, life becomes bigger. Life is easier when all of the sweetness and all of the pain are shared. Now you realize that you must share everything: your time, your drink, and your panic. Everything. This is also true for your happiness, your uncertainty, your dreams, your ups, and your downs. If one person forgets this, the other can serve a glass and a cup of this terrible tasting drink, each drinking half at the same time, doing this over and over again for the rest of your lives. It's far better to drink the panic than to have it drink you. It's far better to schedule it, than to have it visit unannounced. Maybe later in life, or maybe even next week, you will begin to think to yourselves: "If we can share a glass and a cup of something we don't like, then we should also find a beautiful glass and a cup so that we can share a taste of something we do like." This, too, must be shared. Everything must be shared—the bitterness and the sweetness. I now see in my mind's eye both of you offering a toast, clinking your glass and your cup, saying, "Let us share it, this terrible taste, so that in time it will leave room for all the sweet drinks and all the sweet surprises that come from being in love with the whole of life and the whole of each other." Did you know that each of you is a glass and a cup? You're both half full of that awful tasting thing, and you're half full of that sweet tasting thing. Share it all, so that all of it becomes all of both of you. I now pronounce you, Cup and Glass! [With this "marriage" pronouncement, Ilona and Ádám both laugh and weep. The audience also laughs, claps, and cheers]

HILLARY: Congratulations! You just started a new wedding tradition. From now on, in addition to having a champagne toast, there will be a cup and a glass half full of something awful tasting at every wedding, to symbolize that everything must be shared—the sweetness and the bitterness of life. One hundred years from now people will wonder how that tradition got started.

BRAD: Yes! And you have a trip to plan—go find the Kofola. It's wonderful that you both have this mysterious way of attracting all of each other into each other.

HILLARY: Don't forget to make the shop signs.
[Ilona and Ádám nod and stand. Brad, Hillary, and the couple embrace as the audience claps]

The creative therapist can never be reminded enough that the journey of a creative therapy session moves from a small glass to the vast sea. When clients throw the salt of life into a small glass it tastes bad, but when it dissolves into the vast sea, the water tastes refreshing. This also applies to the therapist's own close relationships in which inevitable bitterness must be mixed in the largest container that can be found. If the glass that holds a therapist's relational life is too small, life in and out of sessions will taste like Kofola. If it is held in the vast sea, it is able to change and taste refreshing.

We have a simple prescription for you and your significant other. If you do not have a partner, then do this anyway because you still relate in some way to other human beings and critters you care about. This includes relating to the felt presence of someone who is absent or not yet present. Find the most bitter and worst tasting spice or food powder, paste, or liquid you can find. (Australians offer "Vegemite," along with British "Marmite," Swiss "Cenovis," and German "Hefeextrakt," food pastes made from leftover brewer's yeast extract, if that piques your interest.) In addition to this bitter substance, purchase some fresh honey. Select a time to conduct the ritual of toasting the sweetness and bitterness of your relational life. If you live with someone, each of you should place a tiny bit of "the bitters" in a spoon and then pour some honey over it. Close your eyes and say, "Let us share all the bitterness and sweetness of our lives," and then take the spoonful of this uncommon integrative medicine. Do this every time you find yourself accidentally or purposefully having a disagreement or an upsetting experience with each other. This ritual honors the whole complexity of you both being fully human.

Consider all the bitter and awful tasting experiences that have taken place in all the sessions of your entire therapy life, but don't ponder this for more than fifteen seconds. Imagine it being instantly compressed into a bottle that is as tall as you. Now consider pouring this into the sea. It would immediately dissolve and not be noticeable anymore. Consider this as the bitters of limited therapy being poured into the traditional healer's infinite ocean of mystery. The next time you frustratingly look for a solution to any issue in a session, speak to the ineffable that surrounds it all: "I need a bigger solution—the largest body of water that can dissolve all of therapy and make the session taste better and less bitter."

Throw both the child and adult within you into the vastest ocean of mystery. It is the largest medicine jar that is capable of transforming all bitterness and suffering. Here is found the lifeline that pulls you to the creative lifeboat. The sound of a violin's prayer-song is heard in the sky as a feather tickles a session's softest spot. All of this belongs to your becoming more a part of the fairy tale that enchants a world in need of vast inspiration and creative activation. Welcome onboard the never-ending voyage to change.

10

ELECTRICALLY ORDAINED IN ARKANSAS

Brad conducted a live session at a religious Christian college in Arkansas. He was told that he would see a "famous client" named Stephen, known for likely having been treated by more therapists than any other client in the history of the state. He had been diagnosed with schizophrenia, frequently hospitalized, and intermittently visited a range of outpatient clinics where many students and interns had done their training. Stephen was in his mid-forties and came to the session with his mother and father. Initially watching them talk from a video monitor, Brad heard Stephen talk nonsense about gold mines, two wives, oil fields, and the like. When it was time for Brad to enter the session, on his way he grabbed a five or six-foot-tall potted ficus tree that was sitting in the hall and brought it into the room. Without any explanation he placed it between Stephen and his parents, making it so they had to lean over if they wanted to see each another.

BRAD: Was the world spinning last night?

STEPHEN: Yep.

BRAD: I have seen that you have been keeping it surreal with your parents. You sometimes play a game with them. I assume you are opposed to saying the truth because it would overwhelm others. You can be overwhelming with the way your mind can complexly handle things and express elaborately constructed sentences. It goes past the ability of others who can't keep up with you. I'm going to venture to say that this makes you a man who is an interesting challenge in life.

STEPHEN: Yeah.

BRAD: The question is this: How can you be present, not bored, more awake, and enjoy yourself in a way that won't overwhelm other people while it underwhelms you?

STEPHEN: Easy. I have lots of duties. I am starting a new company across the states. My oil fields are a problem, but it keeps my two wives from seeing each other. I still have that gold mine.

BRAD: Whoa. That's already too much fancy talk. I'm overwhelmed. You gotta keep it simpler and easier for me so I am not overtaken by the power and majesty of your multi-leveled mind. Is it okay if I interrupt you here today whenever I need for you to keep it simple, so I can hear and not be so overwhelmed? You are way above my pay grade and far beyond the cogs of my cognition.

STEPHEN: Sure go ahead.

BRAD: What I want to try to do today is get to what is most essential. By this, I mean what is absolutely most essential about life—your life, your parent's life, my life, and everybody's life.

STEPHEN: OK.

BRAD: If there was one word that would describe why you're on the planet, what would that one word be? What's the one word you are the ambassador for in this lifetime? What word do you think best represents your life purpose?

STEPHEN: The same thing that we each are here for in this life. We are all God's blessed people and the first blessing is to spread the good news.

BRAD: You are an ambassador who is supposed to spread the good news?

STEPHEN: Yes.

BRAD: So, in one word what is the good news?

STEPHEN: Yahweh.

BRAD: Thank you. Now how do you explain Yahweh to someone who says please explain this in a few simple words? Assume they are not an advanced theologian or an ordained minister.

STEPHEN: In just a few words I'd say that we are all created equal, and we are obligated to pray and stay in close contact with our maker, Yahweh. We are to do this through his only son, who was born to the Virgin Mary.

BRAD: Are we here to participate in the creation of life?

STEPHEN: Yes, participate in life.

BRAD: Which is what process?

STEPHEN: The process of creation.

BRAD: [Looking at his parents] Your son just expressed a clear theological understanding of the nature of creation and he expresses it in a way that sounds like a minister or a theologian who knows how to speak to the masses.

STEPHEN: I just talk to the truth.

BRAD: Don't be so modest. I'm saying you can also express things at such a high level that is above other people's ability to understand. You obviously have two means of communication—one overwhelms and the other is as clear as the water in a trout stream.

STEPHEN: I find no problem with this definition. Yes, I do have a problem matching the level of understanding of another person's level of words and comprehension.

BRAD: Mom and Dad, do you hear that he understands his problem and situation?

MOTHER: I have never heard him speak this clearly.

FATHER: It's amazing. To God be the glory!

BRAD: I've been here five minutes and it is clear to me that, as old timers used to say, that your son is too smart for his own good. And this leads to all kinds of issues, confusions, surprises, and drama. When he is able to use words with the kind of precision and caring we just heard, his expression is inspiring. But he also knows how to mentally overwhelm other people. I am going to hypothesize that he thinks that clear expression is only for children or for more simple people like me. And he has assumed that adult talk needs to be more complicated than it need be. He overestimates other people's mental abilities, and this leaves him disappointed with his results.

STEPHEN: Right.

FATHER: I didn't know he was clear like this. What did you put in the water? I have never heard him say anything logical since he was in high school. He's seen so many therapists that every clinic in the state knows him. He's probably taken every medication and has been repeatedly admitted to hospitals because everything he says is complete gibberish. What happened?

BRAD: If I were a five-year-old, he would know how to be clear with me. But if I'm an adult he overshoots my intellectual capacity. I would have to say to you both again, [looking at the parents] that he overestimates the mental capacity of others. He thinks the world is much smarter than it is. Unfortunately, it isn't, and he keeps waiting for other adults to be able to handle language like he can. This has left him very alone and unable to fulfill his mission.

MOTHER: I never would have thought that but when he was a child he spoke to his pets like they were adults and he enjoyed proving to other children that he was smarter by using big words. I never thought anything of it.

BRAD: That is exactly what we are talking about here. Perhaps you forgot to explain to him that others aren't as clever with words as he is and that this is a talent that is both a curse and a blessing.

FATHER: Maybe his words are too big for everyone else's britches! [Laughter]

BRAD: I could not have said it better!

MOTHER: What can we do about this?

BRAD: Stephen, how would you talk to me about what is most important in life? This is all I want to focus on today. What is most essential in life, yours and mine? I have spent a lifetime pondering this question and perhaps today there will be a breakthrough. Before you answer, remember that I won't be able to understand it with big words, complicated logic, and acrobatic metaphor. Please keep it simple because it is a vitally important question for everyone in this room and for those beyond these walls.

STEPHEN: Do your best to understand.

BRAD: Does that mean I should have learned more in school?

STEPHEN: Do your best in every situation.

BRAD: What if I don't want to do my best or I don't know how to do my best?

STEPHEN: Then you are going to have a problem. You will have problems if you don't do your best. All students need to do their best at school and you need to do your best here to learn more about things.

BRAD: [To the parents] I want to put what he said on hold and have you take another a look at it. Do you realize that if I showed a video of the last five minutes to schools across America they would want to hire him as a counselor?

FATHER AND MOTHER TOGETHER: Yeah.

MOTHER: It's a miracle.

BRAD: Did you really experience that?

FATHER AND MOTHER: Yes!

BRAD: This is amazing. I think his mind is so up here [raising his hand up] that he has assumed that children are here [hand lower] and adults are here [demonstrating that adults are higher than children], but most adults should be right down here [moving hand down] not far from being a child.

STEPHEN: Yeah.

BRAD: So, it's as overwhelming to other adults as it is underwhelming to you. I have a weird thought that just popped into my mind. It's nothing I expected to imagine thinking about today. It caught me off guard. It's so unusual that I'd like to share it because I think you might appreciate it.

MOTHER: Well let's hear it.

FATHER: Yep, we are ready.

STEPHEN: Please tell me.

BRAD: What if you walked up a stairwell in the sky or climbed Jacob's ladder? [Brad closes his eyes and lowers his voice, speaking slowly and carefully] I envision you having a rare experience. You are shown or revealed all the mysteries of life. This includes the purpose of life—what is most essential. When you come back to Earth you want to tell everybody, but you know that would be overwhelming and they'd be unable to hear what needs to be said and heard in this world. [Brad opens his eyes]

STEPHEN: It would be an impossible situation.

BRAD: [To the parents] Do you agree? [Both nod yes]

FATHER: Did he have an experience like this?

BRAD: If he did, he shouldn't tell us in a way that would overwhelm us. We'd then miss the important teaching he was assigned to share. In a way, you [looking at the parents] have had this experience. You have a son who is impossible to explain, and you noticed he could speak in advanced ways when he was a boy. You are like Mr. and Mrs. Jacob who both climbed the ladder together to see the sun overhead, but were blinded by the strong rays and unable to see what happened to him. [Everyone laughs]

FATHER: Well I haven't heard it described that way before.

BRAD: That's because the therapists and doctors you take him to speak like him—with way too much jargon and complicated thoughts. They overwhelm everybody with all that medical mumbo jumbo.

MOTHER: That is the truth!

BRAD: [To Stephen] You have a mission and a challenge few people are given. There are a reason and a job you were put on this planet to fulfill. Do you believe what you just told me about what you said your life was all about? I believe you do. Do you?

STEPHEN: I do.

BRAD: I agree that you do. I felt like bringing this tree into the room [pointing to the ficus tree that is in between Stephen and his parents]. I didn't know why. I trusted my inner voice and all I could think is that things are not always what they appear to be. This tree does not know whether it belongs here or not. It just keeps growing. Actually, it's plastic so it is even more mysterious because it wants to appear like it's real when it is not. If I thought too much about the tree and why it's here rather than there, or why it's plastic rather than wood, I'd be overwhelmed. Stephen, how tall are you?

STEPHEN: I am 5 feet and 9 inches.

BRAD: Thank you. Would you please stand next to this tree that doesn't know it's not a tree?

STEPHEN: Sure.

BRAD: Whoa, that is amazing. You are the same height. I actually must tell you the truth. I thought you were at least a foot taller. I had a grandfather who I thought was much taller than he was. There was something about the way he fit in a room that made him seem taller. He commanded attention and he felt bigger than life to me. [To the parents] Maybe you had a grandson and skipped over the son. Maybe that is why he overwhelms—he's too grand.

STEPHEN: May I comment on this?

BRAD: Yes, sir.

STEPHEN: I worked too hard as a youngster and … I became interested in eagles. We've got them here in Arkansas. They migrate in, so you can only see them part of the time.

MOTHER: You can go to Hot Springs to see them.

FATHER: Yeah, along with elks, buffalo, and an animal that looks like an antelope but isn't …

BRAD: Do you know what's interesting about what you all are saying?

FATHER: What?

BRAD: This tree looks like a tree, but it isn't. Your son seems taller than he is like my grandfather appeared, but both were not that tall. And then you mention seeing other special animal sightings that included one that looked like an antelope but wasn't.

FATHER: They look like an antelope. Farmers are having trouble with them because they eat up all of their hay.

BRAD: People always have trouble with critters and people they misidentify. Like your son who is the same height as this tree rather than 1,000 feet tall like a television antenna enabling him to hear too much. Where else did you see critters, you weren't sure what they really were?

FATHER: That's why I wanted to go to Yellowstone.

MOTHER: You wanted to go to Yellowstone, but …

FATHER: Well, we planned the trip but didn't get there. We went off the road at some exit that looked pretty neat. You just kind of said, hey, "Let's go check it out." We ended up in a place called the Tabernacle in the Wilderness. It had a big sign out there. It's a big Catholic Church that was really interesting. Been there since the 1800s. We never made it to Yellowstone.

BRAD: And it looks like your family made another exit off the road and here we are all together surprising one another. Maybe this is another Tabernacle in the Wilderness or maybe its Yellowstone National Park with critters that look like what they aren't. I don't know yet.

FATHER: I never made it to Yellowstone.

MOTHER: But we made it to the Tabernacle in the Wilderness.

BRAD: I have one important question to ask your son. You have witnessed his intelligence and ability to simply and clearly and wisely communicate when he realizes that people are not as smart as they appear to be. This family has a lot of experience discovering appearances that are misleading, taking unexpected turns off the main road, and finding themselves in an unexplored wilderness where things said are, shall we say, mysteriously beyond understanding.

STEPHEN: Ask me.

BRAD: [With a long pause] Would you like to teach Sunday School?

STEPHEN: Yes, I would. Yes.

BRAD: My father and grandfather were country preachers. Let me tell you how my father started.

STEPHEN: Please tell me.

MOTHER: I didn't know you were a preacher's kid.

FATHER: That's great. So, you understand where we are coming from—we are a God-loving family.

BRAD: My father gathered the local dogs and put them in a circle out in the woods. I guess you'd say today that it was his Tabernacle in the Wilderness. He considered this his own hidden church. There he pretended he was preaching to the dogs. He found out that if he sounded sincere and kind and looked like he was going to treat them with a snack, they would pay attention. Otherwise, they walked away as if not a word he said made any sense at all.

STEPHEN: That is awesome and hilarious. [Laughing]

BRAD: My grandmother used to say that is how he learned to teach and preach. "If you can make a dog listen, people will be easy to work with." That's what she would say and then start cackling. She loved repeating that story. And we all loved hearing it.

STEPHEN: I'll be doggone! That makes good sense. It really does! [Laughing]

BRAD: Seriously, Stephen, do you prefer talking to dogs or cats?

STEPHEN: I like cats. I'm fond of cats.

BRAD: Of course you do. A cat is more unpredictable and more impossible and overwhelming. I'm going to take a little break now, get myself a glass of water, and then I'll be back.

Brad goes back to a group of observing therapists, most of them ordained ministers and pastoral counselors. Some mention how shocked and moved they were to see how clear Stephen's talk suddenly became. They had worked with him in their graduate school internship or externship as he was sent to one clinic after another over the years. Several mentioned that the session felt "spiritual" and wondered whether more than therapy was going on. They felt a shift that was mysterious and unexplainable, and Brad asked them to consider how to utilize what they were feeling. He further asked if they would like to personally experience how the room feels from the inside, mentioning that there was a special energy in the room that was quite noticeable. Practically every therapist wanted to feel it firsthand, so a ritual was designed that would enable this exploration to transpire.

[Brad reenters the session room and immediately moves the tree out of the way]

BRAD: We are going to do something that will open a new chapter in your life. My colleagues watching the session in the other room have been touched by what is going on in this room. They would like to enter the room and feel its special atmosphere. Is this fine with the family? [They all nod with enthusiastic approval]

MOTHER: Yes, the room feels like a chapel or someplace special. I feel it.

FATHER: I was going to say the same thing. We took an unexpected turn for sure.

STEPHEN: Are they coming now? I welcome this because this is a special moment.

BRAD: Yes and there is something I'd like you to do for them. Stephen. I want you to give each of them a special blessing. Almost all of them have all taught Sunday School or ministered a church. They would appreciate a sincere blessing from you.

FATHER: Please don't overwhelm them, son.

STEPHEN: I won't. [His father reaches over and shakes Stephen's hand as a sign of this agreement]

BRAD: I'm going to bring in some brothers and sisters who walk with your faith, what you have dedicated yourself to following. As you bless them in the way a child could understand and appreciate, you will be ordained to move on with your life mission. I feel something beyond words at work here so let's not interfere and allow whatever needs to happen.

STEPHEN: Amen!

FATHER: Amen!

BRAD: May good will be amongst us.

STEPHEN: Oh yes!

BRAD: I'll do my best to remember what my father and grandfather would say in this kind of situation. Let all of us ask that this room become a fountain of blessings. Each of these men and women who will come in is in need of a spiritual boost for they too have received the call to minister to the needs of others. I ask that Stephen keep it simple, so all the other children of faith can feel his inner light shine. Let him be neither underwhelming nor overwhelming. Let him be someone focused on helping rather than impressing. May his feet remain on solid ground as his voice provides a sincere tone with spoken words that are felt as true, a medicine to anyone who is down and blue.

STEPHEN: Praise God the creator! I've been a persecuted man and I have felt things that have not been fair. I am often unseen or misidentified. I want all these things to be cleared and made simple so what comes forth is pure.

BRAD: Go on Sunday School teacher! Say it! Go on!

STEPHEN: Let's go! I'm ready for it.

Brad now starts singing a revised version of an old African-American spiritual: "There is a balm in Gilead, to make the wounded whole; there is a balm in Gilead to heal the sick soul; there is a balm in Gilead that makes a man tall as a tree."

STEPHEN: Thank you for that medicine. Thank you.

[At this time around thirty-five preachers and pastoral counselors line up in the hall to enter the room one at a time. The lights are turned off. Stephen gives each of them a short verbal blessing. Some are weeping and others are holding hands. The atmosphere in the room is emotionally strong with a viscerally felt current. At the end, everyone claps in praise]

BRAD: I am going to ask several of the preachers to come and ordain this man to follow his calling. [Three men and two women step forward to provide some appropriate words]

STEPHEN: On the mountain of … [Brad interrupts]

BRAD: You don't have to prove anything, impress, or overwhelm with words. I only want to know if you feel this?

STEPHEN: Oh yes!

BRAD: What do you feel in the air?

STEPHEN: It's strong electricity.

MOTHER: I have never felt anything like this.

FATHER: It's definitely electrical.

STEPHEN: No doubt about it. It's the holy spirit.

BRAD: Hold on to this feeling so it will make your words count. Talk to these pastors with your heart. Talk to my heart.

STEPHEN: Let us be like children in front of the Lord.

BRAD: Thank you.

[The ordaining pastors shake Stephen's hand and congratulate him]

BRAD: Let's put you in front of the tree with your parents at your side.

BRAD: [Kneeling down in front of Stephen] What if I only had one hour left to live. What would you say to me now? Please speak to me as a child in need.

STEPHEN: Know the truth and feel the truth knowing that you accept the truth.

BRAD: Thank you, Stephen! It is your heart that needs to be heard by others not just your highfalutin mind. Just like you did now. Congratulations. I think everyone here is so grateful for your gift that they'd like to also give you a blessing. Don't listen to their words with your mind; listen with your heart and hear their heart express a blessing for you. [Using a melodic tone Brad sings Stephen's formerly spoken line] "Know the truth and feel the truth knowing that you accept the truth."

[Other people reenter the room and whisper a blessing into Stephen's ears and then each leaves the room]

STEPHEN: Thank you so much.

STEPHEN: [To a pastor who kneels in front of him] Grab hold of the Holy Spirit when you realize he is touching you.

BRAD: I felt that! Thank you!

STEPHEN: [To another pastor] Let God touch your life and open your eyes.

PASTORS WHO STAYED IN THE ROOM: Thank you! Amen!

BRAD: [Clapping his hands] I felt that!

FATHER: Son, we love you.

MOTHER: This is a big step for you, Stephen. I love you and will pray for you.

[Brad pulls out a flashlight from his pocket and shines it on Stephen's face]

BRAD: This is all about your being a light and helping other people find the light. Be a light that is a lighthouse rather than a blinding light for others. When others are lost in words, shine the clear light. You will always have a complex mind and complicated speech for those times when it can serve you. But remember there will be other times that need the words children can understand. You must learn to walk with both ways of thinking and speaking. Not just one, but both, each in their right time and place. Do you understand what I am saying?

STEPHEN: Oh yeah.

BRAD: When the mind wants others to know it can overwhelm, then fine, use it wisely. But when it's important for you to help or teach, your mind must produce simple words that shine the truth rather than blind and bind others.

STEPHEN: Be still with them.

BRAD: Be still with them and say simple words. I want you to sit with this experience. I want you to silently pray over this. I want you to even silently sing with this. And think about tonight when you go to bed. Then you can rejoice the day you were electrically ordained in Arkansas.

STEPHEN: God bless you.

BRAD: Bless you, Stephen. I want you to sit in here for a while. [Brad hands him the flashlight] Hold this light and I will soon come back.

[Brad exits. Stephen sits in silence and darkness while holding the flashlight. A few minutes later, Brad returns]

BRAD: Thank you for coming. We all learned a lot today. Don't forget you can practice with the cats if you so choose. Take it one step at a time. Make sure some of the steps have clear and simple words. And then throw in some treats or some surprises from time to time to keep critters on their toes. Explore what happens when you speak simply and do so from the heart. Notice how others will hear and see you differently. You might be seen as having the sight of an eagle, the strength of a buffalo, or the mirage of an illusory antelope, or the height of a tree. You can also be a child of God as easily as you can be an overwhelming man. What's most important is your timing—making sure when it's the time and place to change your speech. Offer what best fits whatever is at hand. People are hungry for clear and wise talk, and people are in great need. Make sure you don't miss them, overwhelm them, or lose your mission. Here's a leaf from the tree so you'll never forget that things aren't always what they seem to be. Go ahead and grow in this life. Stand tall until it's time to sit. Speak until it's time to be quiet. Teach until it's time to learn. Be a son who receives your parent's nurturance until it's time to take care of them. Be a man on a mission until it's time for the next mission. That's it. Go ahead and take the flashlight. You are better prepared to use it than I am.

The most remarkable outcome of this session was voiced afterwards when many in the audience said it was the most powerful spiritual experience they had ever had—that there was an electricity in the room that was felt by the body. Some people were trembling. Several pastors said they realized that they had never directly felt the "holy spirit" before this session.

Brad also felt an electrical current in the room—it was impossible not to feel it. This is what we have felt in healing ceremonies all over the world, no matter the religion or healing way. We have felt it in Africa, Mexico, Chile, the United Kingdom, Hungary, Brazil, and in our home in New Orleans, among many other places. This experience is what is almost always found missing in therapy. The creative therapist allows enough room for it to arrive, something that cannot be forced or willed. But when it comes knocking on the door, the therapy door opens, and the room becomes a place of healing.

Go ahead and get yourself a flashlight and place it by your bed. The next time you wake up in the middle of the night, reach out for it and flash it for a brief second. Immediately ask for a flash to appear in your sessions. Do this while remembering that Milton Erickson once saw a woman client who said she had lived in Phoenix for the last fifteen years and hated every moment of it. Her husband offered her a vacation in Flagstaff, but she refused to go because she preferred to stay in Phoenix and hate it. Erickson told her, while she was in trance, that she should be very curious about why she hates Phoenix and punishes herself so much. There is another thing he told her to be even more curious about: "If you go to Flagstaff for a week you will unexpectedly see a flash of color." She went to Flagstaff with her husband out of curiosity and sure enough she was shocked to see a flash of color. She was so elated that she stayed a whole month in Flagstaff. The flash of color she saw was a redheaded woodpecker going past an evergreen tree. After this trip, she and her husband traveled all over the world and kept looking for and seeing surprising flashes of color.

It's time for you to become more curious about the creative sparks in your therapy and the world around you. Reach for the flashlight and stare off in space toward the direction of Flagstaff or Phoenix. You, too, will someday see a flash, flicker, or spark, or feel a current of electricity or a tingling vibration that will light and excite your session room as well as your world. This is what it means to heal rather than get lost in the spiel that only talks rather than illumines and charges change. If you wish, go find a plastic ficus tree and only glance at it repeatedly without staring. For a second you will think it's real and this experience alone will make you and your therapy both more real and unreal. Or you might get lucky and spot or hear a redheaded woodpecker or a redheaded creative therapist say, "Welcome to your next creative therapy adventure."

11

THE LIGHTNING KING

A middle-aged man, Tom, came to us and said his best friends sometimes called him "King" and that his parents also addressed him with this name. He added that he had numerous middle names as well. After mentioning that he had a desk job and handled a lot of paperwork, we asked him, "Are you the paperwork king?" He answered with a smile, "Yes, I am. The only one."

Tom soon shifted to saying how things had been tough in his life and that he might need a box of Kleenex to get through the session. It was obvious that telling his story would not be a boring rehash but an important performance. We encouraged him to continue. He told the story of how his thirty-year-old son was an alcoholic and that he constantly tried to help him, but that his son recently moved away and left without saying goodbye. We heard how this struggle has been going on for years, and that Tom had gone bankrupt trying to help solve his son's addiction problem. Not only did he want to help his son, he constantly worried about his grandchildren. He mentioned that his son had all the "right tools" to change his life but didn't use them. All of this led to great stress in every part of Tom's life, from work to his marriage. He said he could no longer relax and had even lost the ability to cry. "Nothing seems right" and "I don't want to be strong for everybody else because as the weak ones lean up against me, eventually I'm going to fall. I'm falling now."

HILLARY: We are witnessing an exceptional human being. We both recognize this. There are two things I want to share with you right now. Number one: I bet you've always managed to find yourself in the middle of everything.

TOM: Yeah.
BRAD: You get yourself right smack in the middle of every situation.
TOM: That is right.
HILLARY: At work?
TOM: Yes.
BRAD: With friends?
TOM: Yep.
HILLARY: Everywhere?
TOM: Yep, that's me.
HILLARY: That's must be why you have so many middle names?
TOM: I've got several of them.
BRAD: Yes you do and that's very interesting for someone who's an expert at finding yourself in the middle.
TOM: I hadn't thought that before, but you are right.
HILLARY: The second thing we want to share with you is that I have an intuition that you have a very interesting desk at work. I think there are things on your desk that are probably interesting. Would you say that's true?
TOM: I don't know if they're interesting or not. They may be.
HILLARY: Tell me. What's on your desk?
TOM: A lot of paperwork. [Tom laughs]
HILLARY: What else?
TOM: A computer and a telephone.
HILLARY: Is it all work stuff?
TOM: All work stuff.
HILLARY: Are you permitted to have things on your desk that are non-work items?
TOM: Oh yes.
HILLARY: Do you have a photograph on your desk?
TOM: I have photographs but they're in front of me on another shelf.
BRAD: Is everything on your desk all business?
TOM: Always.
HILLARY: That surprises me. I thought you would have a lot more variety than that.
TOM: Oh, I do have a frog on my desk.
HILLARY: A frog?
TOM: Yes, a frog.
BRAD: That is interesting. Very interesting.
TOM: I collect frogs.
HILLARY: You collect frogs?
TOM: Well, when I was younger, in my 20s, I loved frogs, and I'd get every kind of frog I could find.
HILLARY: "Really!"

TOM: Then everybody started giving me frogs.

HILLARY: Was this interest born when you were in your 20s?

TOM: Yes, that is when it started.

BRAD: How did that happen? Did you wake up one day and spontaneously discover that you loved frogs?

TOM: I don't know. I saw a frog that was interesting.

BRAD: You saw a frog that changed your life?

TOM: I just liked it, so I started collecting different types of frogs.

HILLARY: Do you mean live frogs or figurines?

TOM: Not live ones. Figurines. Then everybody started getting me frogs. My son, wife, and friends brought me frogs.

BRAD: Are we talking about three or four frogs, or thirty frogs?

TOM: We're talking at least thirty frogs at home—inside the house and outside in the yard.

HILLARY: And on your desk is one frog?

TOM: I have one frog on my desk. Actually, I have another frog on my calculator that was given to me by a co-worker two holidays ago.

HILLARY: Really?

TOM: Yes, I actually do have different frogs at work. I have a tadpole frog on my desk. A friend found it in Tahiti. That's why it's on my desk.

HILLARY: Did you find your middle name to be, "Frog"? Are you the Frog Man?

TOM: I know another frog man.

BRAD: You know another frog man?

TOM: He also collects frogs.

BRAD: How'd you meet?

TOM: He worked in another department at work, the one next to mine. One day he walked by my desk and saw my frog. He asked whether I collect frogs? I said, "Yes, a little bit." He then asked me to come look at his office. I had the plain, down to earth, playful frogs. He had fancier frogs.

BRAD: This is so fascinating for many reasons, some of which I'm not even sure I understand. I'd like to know what attracts you to the frogs. Is it how they look, or do you also like how they sound?

TOM: How they look.

HILLARY: Do you like how they sound?

TOM: Not really.

HILLARY: Some people would want to like how they look, and how they sound, and how they feel, and how they touch, because they like it all. But you're okay with just liking how they look. Did you ever handle a frog?

TOM: Not since I was a kid. I don't want them in my hand. My grandkids love them. They pick them up and tote them around all day long.

HILLARY: So, you don't really care about how they sound. You don't want to touch them. But you like how they look enough to become devoted to being a frog man.

TOM: I don't make a big deal out of it.

HILLARY: That's very interesting.

TOM: I mean that I don't go out and buy them. They're given to me.

HILLARY: What I am going to say may sound crazy, but I have to ask it. When something sounds crazy, I have to trust it. Here's my question: What would be the ideal size of frog for you? Let's say you had the perfect frog. What size would it be?

TOM: It would be tiny like a baby frog.

HILLARY: Real tiny?

TOM: I like small frogs.

BRAD: Now let's give it a voice that you'll like. Will it have a male or a female voice?

TOM: A male voice.

BRAD: A male voice. Will it be a child, parent, or grandparent? What age?

TOM: Interesting! I'm not sure. I would say, probably an adult, that is, an adult voice in a small frog.

HILLARY: An adult male voice for a small frog. Would you prefer hearing it sing if it could sing, or just listening to it talk?

TOM: Just listening to it talk.

HILLARY: Would it give you the news every day?

TOM: Yes. I like that. Then I wouldn't have to watch TV every day.

HILLARY: Would it tell jokes?

TOM: Yes, it would have to tell jokes.

HILLARY: Would it tell you the answer to any question that you have in life so that it's like a magical frog?

TOM: No.

BRAD: Fascinating. You just want it to tell you the news. Probably forecast the weather, too. [Tom nods his head in agreement] Do you want the local news or foreign news?

TOM: Local news.

BRAD: Perhaps from time to time would it be okay if it gave you the lottery number?

TOM: Sure, I'll take that, as long as it is the right number.

BRAD: Would this perfect frog be light green or dark green?

TOM: Light green like the color of money. Ha!

HILLARY: Would it have any spots on it or …

TOM: A smooth frog. I do not like warty frogs. They're ugly.

HILLARY: Let's say that the perfect frog that is just the right size with an adult male's voice that can give you the weather, the local news, and occasionally the right lottery number.

TOM: I'd have to keep this to myself.

HILLARY: That's right, everybody would want to steal your frog, so you must be careful. If it were perfect to hold, how would it feel? Would it be warm or cold?

TOM: It would have to be cold.

BRAD: When it's in your hand, do you want it to hop or be still?

TOM: Be still.

HILLARY: Do you want it to move around all over the house or stay in one place?

TOM: Stay in one place.

HILLARY: Do you want it to be predictable or surprise you all the time?

TOM: Surprise me.

HILLARY: This frog sounds exactly like your son.

TOM: Yep, it does, doesn't it?

BRAD: Yes. You've got the perfect frog already.

TOM: Yep, it really does sound like my son. Amazing, huh?

HILLARY: He gives you a lot of news and weather reports.

TOM: Right, that's it.

BRAD: Do you have a frog already in your possession that looks like this?

TOM: Yes, I do.

HILLARY: Is it at home or work?

TOM: It's at home.

HILLARY: Where do you keep it?

TOM: In a bedroom.

HILLARY: Is it right next to where you sleep?

TOM: No, it's in a bedroom across from me—the second bedroom. It used to be our son's bedroom.

BRAD: Have you ever given anyone a frog as a gift?

TOM: No, I've never given anyone a frog for a gift.

HILLARY: Did you ever think about it?

TOM: Everybody's given me frogs for gifts. I haven't thought about giving one to anyone else.

HILLARY: What would happen if you gave a frog to someone you care about?

TOM: I think they would like it.

BRAD: It would be something special?

TOM: Yes, it would.

BRAD: Because they know what it means to you.

TOM: Yes, that's very true.

HILLARY: Are you ready to start therapy? We can now start doing the kind of thing that you can only do in therapy.

TOM: Okay. I'm ready.

HILLARY: If you called your son, and told him that you decided that you were going to become a frog, what would he think?

TOM: He'd think I was crazy. He might really think I'm losing it. He already does.

BRAD: Would he then worry about you?

TOM: I don't think so.

HILLARY: Are you sure?

TOM: He would laugh his butt off and say, "Oh my God! Dad, what have you been drinking?" He is way up here with me. [Tom motions his hand above his head]

HILLARY: What's that mean?

TOM: He does things and says things that I can't even get close to understanding. I can't comprehend it.

BRAD: He's a philosopher?

TOM: He would like to be.

HILLARY: Really?

TOM: Yes, and I never really noticed it until these last two years.

BRAD: Does he use big words when he talks?

TOM: Yep.

HILLARY: Does he read a lot of books?

TOM: He used to read a lot. He graduated with honors in high school.

BRAD: Does he write or only read?

TOM: He does write. He had all kinds of notes on his bedroom wall before he left home. He put up all kinds of sayings.

HILLARY: Like what?

TOM: He used the word "imagine" a lot and the word "anonymous." He'd make poems.

HILLARY: Has he ever commented on your frogs?

TOM: Not that I recall.

HILLARY: What's he think of them?

TOM: I have no idea.

HILLARY: You could call him and ask what he thinks of your frogs.

TOM: He'd probably hang up on me. He is hardheaded and stubborn.

BRAD: Like you?

TOM: Yes. And like my father. Yep, yep.

BRAD: Frogs are stubborn, aren't they?

TOM: He almost died three times. He's been on alcohol and drugs.

BRAD: How about you? Are you someone who's had close calls with death?

TOM: No.

HILLARY: Never?

TOM: I got struck by lightning once.

HILLARY: That's what I'd call a close call.

TOM: My oldest brother calls me "Lightning."

BRAD: Seriously?

TOM: He calls me "Lightning."

HILLARY: We've heard that your life can change after you get hit by lightning. Sometimes people all of a sudden get new abilities that no one can explain.

TOM: It happened when my son was small.

HILLARY: He was there?

TOM: Yes, he was there when it happened.

BRAD: He saw you get hit?

TOM: I was talking on the phone. My son saw it. He can remember it like it was yesterday. He actually has the capability to be caring, loving, help with everything, and even take charge.

BRAD: Maybe those are the kind of people lightning likes to strike.

TOM: Well, if it struck him, I'd hope it would shake some sense into him.

HILLARY: Like it struck you.

TOM: Yes. It did; it got me. It put me down for a while.

HILLARY: For how long?

TOM: I was physically down for about a month. Then I started coming back.

HILLARY: So you were really hit?

TOM: I was really hit, yes.

BRAD: How old were you when it struck?

TOM: I was twenty-four years old.

HILLARY: About the time you started liking frogs?

TOM: Yes.

BRAD: That's an interesting connection.

TOM: I guess you could say that. I didn't have any frogs in my home until after that lightning hit me.

HILLARY: You were struck by lightning, it wiped you out for a month, you came back to life, and then all of a sudden, you love frogs. Wow!

TOM: That is exactly what happened!

BRAD: Are you able to influence people? Do you have an influence on people?

TOM: I would hope so.

HILLARY: [In a teasing manner] I'm not talking about your son because sons are impossible if you're their dad. I'm thinking of other people. Are you a person who has influence?

TOM: I would think so. Yes.

HILLARY: Perhaps it is not the case that you're so much in the middle of things. You just sort of attract all the charge.

TOM: Exactly. How, how do I stay out of it?

BRAD: I think it's your destiny.

TOM: You think it's my destiny?

BRAD: I mean that lightning came looking for you. You attracted its charge.

TOM: I actually saw it. That's the weird part about it. I saw lightning coming straight down toward me.

HILLARY: You saw it?

TOM: It was a storm and I was standing at the back door, talking to a friend at work on the telephone. As I was looking out the back window, I saw lightning far off, coming straight down. The next thing I know, I'm on the floor.

HILLARY: That's amazing. This is like the story of your life. I'm sure you see the storm brewing around you all the time—whether it's at work or in your family. You see it brewing, you see it building, and then you see the lightning bolt coming. It hits you every time.

TOM: Totally! Why is this?

HILLARY: You just keep getting struck by lightning.

TOM: I do. I keep getting struck by lightning all the time.

HILLARY AND BRAD TOGETHER: Wow!

TOM: Is that a good thing or a bad thing?

HILLARY: It's more a mysterious thing.

TOM: Really?

HILLARY: Not everybody gets struck by lightning. This is what happened in your life. Again, it's not that you're in the middle even though it may appear that way. It is more accurate to say that you are a lightning rod.

TOM: Do I need to walk around with a piece of …

BRAD: Maybe you want to be a better conductor.

TOM: I am a take-charge person. I like to do things the right way. I like to make sure they're done the right way.

BRAD: Do you know how to shoot lightning?

TOM: No.

HILLARY: You only know how to get hit by it?

TOM: Yes, I know how to catch it. It only takes one time to learn that.

HILLARY: You are the Lightning King.

TOM: Here I am.

HILLARY: Not just a king. You're *the* Lightning King.

TOM: I think so.

BRAD: When you give your son and others instruction, do you point your finger at them?

TOM: I intentionally try not to do that because that is a behavior that was inherited by my sisters. They point with their finger too much.

HILLARY: It's probably a good thing that you didn't use that finger because it wouldn't surprise me to find out that you have a little extra bolt of something that others don't have. It might be too strong for others to handle. I think it would be good for you to draw a little crown on the tip of your pointing finger. It's time that you wear your crown. Whenever the occasion, whether it's with your son, or other friends or workers, remind them that you were struck by lightning. Tell them, "All I can say is that I was struck by lightning and I am still alive." You don't have to explain anything; simply say that. Whenever you say this, it will be like shooting lightning as you say it. Anyone who's been struck by lightning and remains alive to talk about it makes everyone get a tingle when they hear it! It's such a rare thing. There are all kinds of stories about people who change after they are hit by lightning. Sometimes they gain powers or receive an intuitive a gift, or simply find themselves different. In your case, you started liking frogs.

TOM: Why can't I just be normal? Why can't I stay out of the middle?

BRAD: You will never be normal. You were struck by lightning.

TOM: Yes, that's what they told me.

HILLARY: You were struck by lightning. Perhaps it's time you learn to enjoy it as opposed to being concerned about it.

TOM: I tried to learn to enjoy it.

HILLARY: You are the indisputable Lightning King. It's time you tell other people who you really are. And don't you ever forget it. There are many interesting ways of communicating this to others. You could be having a casual conversation about the weather or about the news and just throw in a reminder, "Don't forget, I was struck by lightning."

BRAD: Or you could be in an argument, and then suddenly announce, "Don't you forget, I was struck by lightning, and I'm still alive." When you get the courage, you could start adding something that's going to really be a shock, like a lightning bolt of surprise. Then you might say, "Don't forget, I was hit by lightning, and ever since that moment, I have a lot of frogs." That would really shock someone.

TOM: Yes, it probably would.

HILLARY: It would be like sending them a lightning bolt, a little bolt. If they know you, they're going to think, "Yep, he has those frogs" and they're going to wonder, "What in the world does all that mean?"

BRAD: Somebody might ask you, "Is there something meaningful about those frogs?" You should tell them the truth. Say, "There must be a special meaning, but I don't know what it is. It just happened after the lightning."

TOM: It is weird how that happened. It is really weird.

HILLARY: It is weird.

BRAD: Your life is weird.

HILLARY: It truly happened to you. You were struck by lightning and ever since you've in the middle of everything. You're the lightning rod. You can see the storm brewing including all the conflicts that happen to people in your home and at your workplace. When it builds and builds, you can see it coming. Then it comes straight at you and you get zapped. You get up all over again and you think that you don't want to do this anymore. But you get up and there you are, surviving another bolt all over again.

TOM: On to the next one.

BRAD: You wait around for the next lightning bolt and the next frog. I wonder how your life would be different if you owned who you truly are? Say to yourself over and over again, "Here's my crown, I'm the Lightning King." Do it to build up enough confidence to shoot some bolts into others who need it. If you feel like another person might benefit from a little shock in their life and that it would be good for them, send them a bolt. Tell them about the lightning and the frogs that followed. Say whatever you want about the frogs. "Ever since I was hit by lightning, the frogs came into my life."

TOM: It's true about the frogs. I can't get rid of them. After the lightning hit me, they came to my house like crazy.

BRAD: Do you mean there's an infestation of frogs everywhere around you?

TOM: Yes, live frogs started showing up everywhere around me.

HILLARY: That's unbelievable.

TOM: It is really the truth.

BRAD: If you own your crown and tell people this truth, it's going to be like lightning hit them. I'm in shock right now realizing that I have met the Lightning King who reigns over a kingdom of frogs. They're all around you.

TOM: It is totally amazing, isn't it?!

HILLARY: This is who you are. As soon as you remind others, you'll know how to act. My feeling is that something will start to move in your life. It may take place in your relationship with others, with life itself, with lightning, or with the frogs.

TOM: Why is it that when I try to work things out, or when I try to be happy, jolly, and come to work dancing so to speak, I get kicked because nobody wants to hear it, and nobody wants to see it? Then it bothers me all day.

HILLARY: You started this session, telling us that you have several middle names, and now you have another name. In some unexplainable way it seems you have been trying to find the name that tells others who you are. But now you can crown yourself the Lightning King. It is time for you to remind others that you were struck by lightning and survived, and then the frogs came into your life. If you do this wisely, people are going to pay attention to everything you say. Do you hear what I'm saying?

TOM: Yes, I hear you.

BRAD: We are very serious.

TOM: I know, I know.

HILLARY: The wonderful thing about all this is that we're just holding a mirror up to you.

TOM: I know, but why does everybody think that I need to take control when I really don't. I just want to help.

BRAD: You can't find out until you own your crown and accept who you are.

TOM: You mean accepting the fact that I am the Lightning King?

BRAD: Yes.

TOM: I have to own who I am?

HILLARY: Crown yourself.

TOM: I give myself credit for that.

HILLARY: Give yourself credit for what happened to you. You survived the bolt and then the frogs came. The frogs are on your desk, they are in your home, and they're all around your yard.

TOM: They're on my porch. They're even in my flower pots.

BRAD: It's like the universe is saying, "You're on pause until you finally get who you are." No one is paying attention to you in the way that you expect because you are on pause. The second you accept your crowning truth; your life will go forward.

TOM: As soon as I accept it.

HILLARY: Own it, celebrate it, and announce it.

TOM: Is this why I feel the way I do?

HILLARY: All we know is that you are stuck; you are on pause. When you are on pause you can't get an answer. Push "play" and move your life forward.

TOM: That's why I feel like I'm in a rut? And can't get out?

HILLARY: You are on pause.

TOM: What do I do about my son?

BRAD: Find out what the Lightning King will do. You're hopeless.

TOM: I'm hopeless, but the King knows.

HILLARY: Yep, you are hopeless because the Lightning King is on pause.

TOM: That's funny, very funny.

HILLARY: When you're lightning is in motion, anything can happen.

TOM: It's funny because I've recently been thinking that I want to unleash myself. That's why I came here, and these are words I used for myself.

BRAD: We're inviting you to just press play—so you can move forward.

TOM: So, if I want to wear a crazy tie or get a different haircut …

HILLARY: I don't know. We'll have to wait until the Lightning King shows up. He'll know.

TOM: I've been really kind of wanting to unleash.

HILLARY: Notice that the Lightning King survived. And that's when the surprise came—the frogs showed up.

TOM: They did.

HILLARY: You should write these words down. Take a piece of paper and write out: "I am the Lightning King, with a kingdom of frogs." Then draw a crown on your finger, start telling others who you are, and find that you are no longer on pause, because you have pushed the play button. The emphasis here is on play. Isn't that interesting? When you want to move things forward, it's play. Push play and play. Your life is fascinating. It's been a pleasure meeting you.

TOM: Thank you, thank you. I appreciate it.

Session 2

TOM: I guess you can see I am not that upset this week. [Tom is smiling and has a new flashy red tie]

HILLARY: You came flying in, didn't you?

TOM: Last week I felt better when I left. I felt a lot better. That really helped me.

BRAD: How are things with your family?

TOM: Everything's basically the same with my son, but I'm letting go of the things that I used to do. I really don't want to take care of everybody or worry about my son as much as I have done. Remember when we talked last week about how much I like the frogs?

HILLARY: Yes.

TOM: Well, my best friend come over Sunday and brought me a statue of a frog to put around my pond. It is an old metal frog.

HILLARY: You are the King after all.

TOM: I also crowned myself King this week.

HILLARY: It shows. Congratulations!

TOM: On Friday, when I got off work, I went home and was all by myself. I enjoyed it. Saturday morning, I got up and I also enjoyed myself. I felt like I didn't have to cater to anybody or do anything for anyone else. I have never done that before.

HILLARY: This may sound weird, but I have an unusual question to ask you. Now that you are a king, I think it is time for this question: "Do you know why the birds sing?"

TOM: No.

BRAD: Do you know why lightning struck you?

TOM: No.

HILLARY: Do you know why the goldfish swim?

TOM: No.

BRAD: We would like for you to think about these questions. How can you possibly understand why any human does what they do if you don't understand why the birds sing or why goldfish swim or why lightning struck you or why the frogs come to you?

TOM: True. Thank you, thank you. That's good. Nobody knows why. I've asked myself that so many times.

HILLARY: Now it is time to tell you something very important. We know something about you. This is what we know: You have lightning inside you.

TOM: I've been told that before.

BRAD: I bet you have been told that. You do have the lightning inside of you. But somehow you haven't figured out how the lightning inside of you and the unleashed "no" inside of you can be used in other parts of your life.

TOM: Right.

HILLARY: You can say, "I know things have happened to me in my life that are beyond explanation. I know life itself is beyond explanation, including what's happened to my son. I got struck by lightning and he got struck by alcohol and drugs. I got hit by sky lightning and he got hit by white lightning. He doesn't know why and neither do I." These things happened, and you still have the lightning inside of you. You don't have to be struck like before. You can ask yourself, "I, the King of Lightning, brought the frogs forth. What can I do with the things in my life that could use some lightning?" We have an idea for you.

TOM: Excellent.

BRAD: We see that you wear a gold cross around your neck. Are you a spiritual person?

TOM: Yes, I would say that I definitely am.

HILLARY: Do you believe there are mysteries bigger than anyone's ability to understand?

TOM: Absolutely.

HILLARY: And that there is a sacred aspect of life that looks after everything?

TOM: That's true.

BRAD: This is true for the smallest bird that flies in the sky and its true for the goldfish and the frogs—everything and everyone is important. Every single flaw also has a special reason for its season in life … Anything that happens, whether we think it's good or bad, is more important than what we can understand, and is part of a bigger plan.

HILLARY: Sometimes it's sunny and at other times it rains. Sometimes you get struck by one kind of lightning and at other times you get hit by another kind of lightning. Do you ever feel that you can almost remember what that lightning felt like? Do you ever just think about it and then feel a jerk inside your body?

TOM: Yes! Definitely.

HILLARY: In that way, the lightning keeps striking you.

TOM: Bounces me back.

HILLARY: Bounces you back.

TOM: Jerks me back.

HILLARY: You get jolted. You can't be authentically jolted by lightning in the way it happened to you and then be free of it. You keep on jolting. Thinking about it, dreaming about it, daydreaming about it, considering it, just spontaneously remembering it, brings it back. You can't stop getting jolted.

TOM: Yep, that's how it is.

HILLARY: That's an extraordinary thing.

TOM: It truly is.

HILLARY: You shall forever be jolted by this bolt.

TOM: It's something you never can forget.

BRAD: Can you describe how it looked when you saw it in the sky?

TOM: I remember how it looked when I saw the sky. There was a dark cloud and lightning was coming straight down.

HILLARY: Did it zigzag or come straight down?

TOM: It came straight down.

BRAD: It had no doubt that you were its target?

TOM: Apparently so.

HILLARY: It just went straight for you?

TOM: Yes, it did. The next thing I know, my friends were there taking me to the hospital.

HILLARY AND BRAD TOGETHER: Wow!

TOM: I guess I want to be, and I need to be jolted every now and then.

HILLARY: Of course you do. That lightning made it possible for you to be jolted every time you think about it. Every time it comes back to you, it gives you a little jolt.

[Brad brings his chair closer to Tom and sits directly in front of him. Leaning forward, he reaches out to shake his hand. Brad voices his words gently, with a musical tone]

BRAD: "Wouldn't it be something if you could reach out and shake the hand or hold the hand of someone else whenever you felt the need? Let's imagine someday in the future, maybe 30 years from now, or maybe 30 days from now. There you are reaching out to hold the hand of a grandchild. Or maybe you reach out to hold the hand of someone else. Then you say, "I just want to hold your hand and tell you about the time I got hit by lightning." As you're doing this, you recall the time you were looking out the window and saw that lightning.

HILLARY: You then say, "I was looking outside the window, and all of a sudden I could feel some electricity in the air. I could feel something was about to happen. I knew it. I had a sixth sense at that moment that something unexpected was about to intervene. All I could see was the dark cloud and then all of a sudden, straight for me came that lightning!"

[Brad's hand gently vibrates Tom's clasped hand as Hillary speaks. Both Hillary and Brad's voices are more lyrical and musical, and Tom enters a trance]

BRAD: As you imagine yourself telling that story in the way that only you know how to express it, you remember it and then all of a sudden you feel the jolt.

HILLARY: And when you jolt, you give them a little jolt.

[Brad gives Tom's hand a little jolt]

TOM: I felt it. [Tom nods]

BRAD: Do you hear what we're saying? This is an old-fashioned way of talking about your electricity. You can talk about unexplainable mysteries including being an attractor of lightning and frogs and all kinds of unexplainable things.

HILLARY: You can even talk about what makes it rain. You can also talk about the recharge of life and how things unexpectedly change. You can build-up so much excitement that you feel like all of a sudden there's going to be a bolt. Right?

TOM: That's right.

HILLARY: I bet you can find a way to charge your memory and talk about it, so you can hold somebody's hand and say to those you care for, "You know one day I was struck by lightning. I'm the King of Lightning. Every once in a while, I can just remember it and it strikes me again. I feel a jolt inside of myself. What I'd like to do is share this jolt because it's not fair for me to keep it all inside myself."

TOM: I understand what you are saying.

HILLARY: This is what we want you to do. We want you, as best as you can, to take a piece of paper and draw that lightning bolt. We don't know whether you're going to show it as narrow or wide. We don't know if you're going to use dark paper and make it white, or whether you're going to use white paper and color it yellow, purple, green, or whatever. Do you know whether it was blue or white, or some other color? Do you remember?

TOM: It was a white streak of lightning.

HILLARY: Maybe you need a dark piece of paper with some white lightning. We want you to carry this image of lightning around with you every day if the week. Every time you're in a situation where you think you ought to be able to say no to someone or you think that another person could use a jolt of your lightning, do what we're now going to tell you.

BRAD: In that moment pull out your piece of paper and just look at it. Stare at it and remember the day when lightning struck. Say to yourself, 'There was a day in my life when the clouds got dark and it looked scary outside. I wondered about the safety of my family. I hoped my children wouldn't be hurt 'cause anything can happen in a treacherous storm. As I looked out the window and as I stood in front of my family, that lightning came straight at me and gave me a jolt." As you remember and say this to yourself, allow yourself to experience a jolt. Then put the drawing back in your pocket or purse. If you need to, step out of the room to do it. You can even run outside.

HILLARY: Do this every single time you're in an occasion where you are not sure about what to do, like "What do I need to say to my son?" or "How can I understand even though I know I can't understand it?"

BRAD: When you need to be struck by lightning or notice somebody else who needs to be struck by lightning, do this procedure.

HILLARY: Know that every time you do this, you're going to be charging that bolt. The drawing itself is going to get charged. If you did this five times in a day, it would receive five charges. If you did it 15 times, there would be 15 charges. Now here's your big assignment: After it has been charged for at least three days, we want you to put this lightning bolt underneath your pillow and sleep on it.

TOM: Okay, I will. [Tom nods with enthusiasm]

HILLARY: If it ever needs more charging, you take it out and charge it. If it's sufficiently charged and you have put enough of yourself into that drawing, it will do something to you. It might say, "I'm going to visit you in a dream." Do you believe that?

TOM: It's possible.

BRAD: With you, anything is possible. You could be struck by lightning again in the dark, but this time when your eyes are closed during a dream.

TOM: Could be.

HILLARY: That's something.

TOM: It sure is. That would be something.

HILLARY: We also know that you could be struck in the middle of the night while you're asleep in a dream that you just don't remember.

TOM: I'm ready.

HILLARY: You may wonder whether you got struck while you were asleep, unless you're lucky enough to remember it.

TOM: Or unless I feel something different the next day.

HILLARY: You might wake up and feel something different and if you do, you're going to say, "I was struck by lightning." Or something unexpected might happen the next day and then you will know that lightning got you the night before.

TOM: Yep. Let me tell you what I did last week about my grandkids. When I picked them up from daycare, instead of bringing them home with me, I took them to their parent's house. I had no second thoughts about it and I didn't feel bad about it. When I got home, my wife asked, "Where's the grandkids?" I said, "I took them to their daddy's house." She asked, "Why?" I said, "Well, that's where they live and it's time for their parents to get real." I left it at that.

HILLARY: That's fabulous. I think that your lightning is already doing its job. The Lightning King, the man who brought forth the frogs, will always have lightning inside of him. He is going to be hit more often, especially as that inner bolt is charged. You, Tom, are going to be surprised more often about the things that you do with everyone in your life.

TOM: I think that is true.

HILLARY: A song just rushed into my head. It's a famous old popular song. I don't know why, but it just flooded into me. This time I heard it with different lyrics. Maybe I got struck by a little bit of your lightning. I want to sing it. I don't know if that sounds strange, but may I sing you this song?

TOM: Sure! [Tom smiles]

BRAD: The King needs an honoring song.

HILLARY: I'm going to sing it now [Hillary sings some improvised lyrics to the tune of *Close to You*]: "Why do frogs, suddenly appear, every time, you are near? Just like lightning, they long to be, close to you. Why do you, find yourself in the middle, of so many, people's problems? Because, just like lightning, people long to be, close to you. La la da da da. Lightning King." Sing it with me, please somebody. "La la da da da, Lightning King."

BRAD: [Brad joins in playing the piano and singing] "La la da da da, Lightning King."

TOM: That's pretty cool.

BRAD: Bravo, you're becoming a musical. I would say that anyone who has been struck by lightning, attracts the frogs, and has a life like yours, is going to inspire someone to create a musical.

TOM: Yes, I think so. Well, Hillary just made me a musical.

BRAD: Yes, she just did. You are a musical.

TOM: Why is it that I'm so attracted to people with problems?

HILLARY: [Singing] Because they long to be, you long to be, close to them.

BRAD: Exactly.

TOM: Yes, they do.

BRAD: You lightning bolt, you. Do you understand the task at hand? Are you ready to draw the lightning bolt?

TOM: Yes, I will draw the lightning, carry it with me, and keep charging it.

BRAD: Yes.

TOM: And putting it underneath my pillow.

HILLARY: Yes. Notice when you wake up if you were hit.

TOM: I'm also going to keep drawing a crown on my finger.

HILLARY: Excellent! It would also be nice if you could find a record or CD of that song "Close to You."

TOM: I already have it at home. I will play it tonight! Actually, I just started listening to 70s music recently and that includes the Carpenters.

HILLARY: Really?

TOM: Yes, I'm not sure why, but I started liking it.

BRAD: The universe is lining itself up for all these things to be on your platter, just when you need them.

TOM: So it's like the old saying, "things happen for a reason."

HILLARY: Yes! And it gave you the reason. Listen closely: "La la da da da. Lightning King."

TOM: Okay! [Smiling]

HILLARY: See you next week.

TOM: Thank you for the song.

Session 3

HILLARY: How's the weather?

TOM: I was quite a show this morning. You all missed it. I went to work, walked in, turned on my computer, went to the restroom, and then I looked down and saw that I had on two different shoes. Not just two different colors, but two different shoes.

BRAD: Amazing!

HILLARY: Extraordinary! What a shock! What a bolt!

TOM: I went back to my office and I sat there wondering what I should do. Do I just carry on? Or do I go home and fix it?

BRAD: That's sort of like the question of your life.

TOM: Yes. I fixed it, but in a different way. I went to the store and got some new shoes.

HILLARY: Wild! Shocking! Another bolt!

TOM: But only after I made everybody laugh at work!

HILLARY: Awesome! You brought lightning to your workplace.

TOM: I sure did. It was quite fun. We had a ball with it.

BRAD: We want to celebrate that quality of your life tonight. You have had extraordinary experiences that none of us have ever heard of before we met you. We're convinced there's never been a human being like you. Once upon a time you looked out the window and saw a storm brewing. You saw that a lightning bolt was not uncertain about where it wanted to go. It went straight to you. You were knocked out. Perhaps you went somewhere. Who knows? When people get struck by lightning, some people say that you can go to heaven and see the light. I don't know. Maybe they go to the deepest parts of themselves. It's beyond understanding. Remember that the only explanation for you has to be sung: "La la da da da. Lightning King."

HILLARY: When you came back, the world was different. The frogs came to you, sang to you, and honored you. The lightning brought more frogs into your life. What's even more fascinating is that the lightning never went away. Every time you think about what happened that day, you still get a jolt. That is a remarkable gift. If you always carry a lightning bolt, like your drawing of that lightning, and keep it charged, you are ready for anything.

TOM: I did that. I drew it and I kept it with me. When my grandkids saw it, they took it home with them.

HILLARY: That's wonderful! You should get them to draw other ones, teach them how to charge it, and tell them why you're doing it. Tell them they can have their own custom-made bolts. All of you can do this together. You can also charge each other's bolts.

You can say, "Here I've charged this one, so you can carry it. Did you charge yours for me?" That would be a fun thing.

TOM: Yes, it would be.

BRAD: When the lightning came, it marked you. It said, "I'm pointing to this one, and he's going to get a charge." When you resurrected and came back, you were in a different world. The frogs came to you because they recognized you were no longer the same man.

HILLARY: Although life is still going to be filled with challenges and dark clouds, you have the lightning inside. If you keep it charged, it will empower you and enable you to surprise yourself. You can even look down and see two different shoes on. I wouldn't be surprised if this kind of thing will continue to happen as long as you charge your lightning.

TOM: Nothing like that ever happened before at work. This was the first time.

HILLARY: We have a gift for you tonight.

TOM: Oh really!

HILLARY: We're here to celebrate your life. You have inspired us to put your life to music. It's our way of celebrating the mystery that's inside of you and is now circulating through your family. You all have access to something that others don't. You just have to use it. You have to keep it charged. Let it surprise you and let it come out. Unleash more bolts. You did just that this morning, didn't you?

TOM: Oh yes, I sure did!

BRAD: It's interesting because this was the first time you used your lightning in this way and it changed your workplace. There you were changing the atmosphere surrounding the way people relate to each other. Amazing, isn't it?

TOM: Yes, it absolutely was.

BRAD: Please close your eyes now as we sing you a song and tell you the fairy tale that is the truth of your life. [Keyboard music begins in background as Brad continues speaking and singing, while playing] I have a story to tell. It's going to sound like a fairy tale, but it's a miracle because it's true. There was a man who cared a lot about everything and everyone. He cared so much that he always found himself in the middle of it all. Then one day it started to look like it was going to rain. Things looked dark . . . A storm began to brew and before you knew it, he saw a lightning bolt coming straight at him. Yes, that lightning struck him down and knocked him out. Miraculously he came back. That's when our tale really begins, because at that time something miraculous and unexplainable took place. The frogs came looking for him. When they sang, they were saying to him, "You're the King of Lightning. You bring the storm and deliver the rain. King of Lightning, we're here to stay." The frogs know what it is to be alive. They know there's a mystery to each and every day. No matter what kind of problem, suffering, or storm comes our way, they know it's not easy being green. And they know it's not easy being full of lightning.

[The formerly improvised music changes to the popular song, *It's Not Easy Being Green*]

HILLARY: [Singing] It's not easy, the frogs say, being the king. Just like us, it's not easy being green, and knowing how to be ordinary after you're struck by lightning. Because people just pass on by and don't do the simplest things they should do to help them get along. But we say to you, green is the color of spring, and green can be so friendly, and green can be big like an ocean or important, like a mountain or tall like a tree. Lightning King, life is green, and so are frogs, and so are you. So, every time, you wonder why, why wonder, wonder why I am green like you. Know it's beautiful and I think it's what you ought to be, a Lightning King.

[The music returns to an improvisation that is a melodic mix of excerpts from *Close to You* with the former tune]

BRAD: [Singing while continuing to play the keyboard] Why do the frogs come to you? Why oh why did the lightning strike you down? Why are you in the middle of everything? Why? They long to be close to you. Close to the magic of being green and being alive and knowing there's more than why. There's more than why so why ask why?

[The music now becomes the song, *Close to You* again, as Brad and Hillary both sing]

Why do swans fall out of the sky? Every time, you walk by, just like lightning. They want to be, close to you. On the day that you were struck, the angels got together and decided to create a dream come true. So, they sent a lightning bolt, it struck you down, when you arose, then they all came to you. This is why all the frogs in town, follow you all around. Just like lightning, they want to be close to you.

HILLARY: [With a strong vibration in her melodic tone] Now the lightning is inside of you. Charge it. Remember how you arose after the storm. You finally stood up and said, "I'm going to live again. Now I have the lightning inside of me." This was the cost of being alive with a big heart. It makes everything want to be close to you. Like the lightning, everyone wants to be close to you. Just like the frogs, they want to be close to you. Just like life, it longs to be close to you. Just like you, you long to be close to you. People at work and grandchildren and children at home, they long to be close, close, close to you.

BRAD: Thank you Lightning King. You're the fairy tale that's close to us. Don't bother with another kind of why—everyone just wants to be close to you. You are the Lightning King. Wear your crown and share the bolts. You know what to do. Charge that inner mystery bolt every time you don't know what to do. Let it build up inside. Like lightning, like the frogs, like the green of life—this is unexplainably true."

TOM: How about that! Thank you!

HILLARY: We mean this: Inside of you, the lightning is always ready to act.

TOM: You're right!

BRAD: No matter how old you get; the lightning will remain inside of you. If you remember to charge it, it will be ready to strike in all kinds of interesting, surprising, fascinating, inventive, creative, and beautiful ways.

HILLARY: You might think about something you've never imagined before. That lightning is always going to bring a surprise. It's going to charge the room and change the atmosphere.

TOM: It sure is.

HILLARY: Yes, it sure is. No matter what happens, no matter how often you think you ought to ask why, all you have to do is charge the bolt and wait for it to strike.

TOM: And watch it strike.

BRAD: Yep, that's right.

TOM: Thank you! This is very good. I couldn't have done that musical about my life if I tried. I'm so happy I inspired you to do it!

BRAD: Exactly! Your lightning struck again.

TOM: Yep.

HILLARY: These songs will never be the same.

TOM: I won't ever be the same.

HILLARY: We'll listen whenever the frogs sing and think of you, the crowned Lightning King.

You may not have been physically struck by lightning, but we are sure that you have been surprised by many a storm. Life has likely already sent you all kinds of lightning bolts and thunder rolls that knocked you out or took the wind out of your sail. Perhaps it was falling in love, the birth of a child, the homecoming of a lost friend, a close call with death, or being told your learned therapy is more dead than alive. Hold on to those memories and help them charge your life.

Regard the creative leap each session needs as no more complicated than a frog in action. In other words, when you have trouble speaking on behalf of change, just know there's a frog in your throat that wants to leap. If it helps, fill your room with more than one frog figurine. Wood, metal, ceramic, plastic, clay, or paper—it matters not the material form. It's the leap it helps inspire that determines whether a session sings or croaks. Go ahead and bring more frogs to your room so every small bottle feels closer to the creative pond.

For sure, draw a creative therapy lightning bolt. Make several—one for your pocket, wallet, or purse and another to hang on the wall or dangle from the ceiling that is hung low enough for others to accidentally get hit by it. Charge it every time you feel stuck and wish for something to recommend when others seriously ask for help during a creative dry spell of life. There are many memories that can reawaken and recharge your therapy heart as you remember what it is to feel truly alive. The lightning lives inside of you as strongly as it lives inside of Tom. Charge it and make sure it is ready whenever a session requires a bolt of energized inspiration. Do so whether or not you know why the birds fly, or why the frogs sing, or why Tom was struck by lightning. You don't have to provide an explanation, interpretation, or any hesitation to strike when it comes to being the lightning of change that helps others find a more magical life.

12

OUR LOVE IS HERE TO STAY

In Budapest, we met with Mari and her husband, Miklós, a distinguished and successful man who recently had been told by his medical doctor that he had a terminal illness with less than a year to live. Miklós made clear that he was a skeptical Communist and agnostic, with no belief that anything could help him now. He declared he was just an "ordinary man" who was worried about his wife's forthcoming grief and what could be done to help prepare her for the future. At first, we asked what they might do if they only had a week to live, especially how they might surprise each other with experiences they would never imagine doing. For instance, we asked if they would consider jumping out of an airplane with parachutes. Mari responded that she was being treated for phobias and she could never do this. It was far too frightening to even imagine.

We then asked what they would say to each other if they found out that they only had one hour left to live. To our surprise, they mentioned that this situation had already happened. The previous month Miklós took Mari for a surprise getaway to Italy. When they were on the plane ready to take off, the engine caught fire and they feared they would both be killed. He discovered that all he wanted was to rescue her and that he didn't care if he died trying.

BRAD: Is there anything that you could do today do that would surprise each other?

MARI: [Pauses to think] Everything he does surprises me, because to me he has a very unusual approach to life. I have always been surprised at the way he makes decisions and lives his life. He has never paid any attention to what others say about him and he has always lived how he wanted to live. I care much more than he does about what other people think and give much more importance to meeting others' expectations. He is not this way.

BRAD: If you told him, "I fell in love with the non-ordinary you," that would be a shock to him because he thinks, as he mentioned before, that he is ordinary. In a way, you are in love with the man he doesn't know. Maybe you should introduce him to this other man.

MIKLÓS: I still don't believe it. I am only ordinary.

BRAD: For your entire marriage, he never knew you were in love with a non-ordinary man, because he thinks he is someone else. Very interesting. Maybe he needs a new mirror, because his mirror is broken. What if right now—because you never know, you could walk out of here and get hit by a bus—you tell him this truth again? Why don't you tell him, "I'm in love with a non-ordinary man, and that man is you."

MARI: [Mari laughs and turns to Miklós] You know that—I have told you that before.

MIKLÓS: But I know that this doesn't really fit reality.

BRAD: You know what I think? You need to show her that you are the man she fell in love with, so for the rest of her life she'll know this love was true and real. What is needed right now is some non-ordinary expression from each you to one another. If it makes sense, it's too ordinary. If it doesn't make sense, it's not ordinary. I know right now it's too much for you to jump out of a burning airplane.

I think the first step of being not ordinary right now is that the two of you should immediately go buy a toy airplane. [They both laugh] Go right now, today. If one of you says to the other, "this doesn't make sense," then you must do it. This isn't something for you to think about, it's something for you to do. Although you have many years together already, you are still both children. This is the way life is. So, maybe you should go to the toy store as if you are both ten years old.

MIKLÓS: I don't understand what this is supposed to change or do for us.

BRAD: Perfect. That's the reason to do it. It makes no sense.

MIKLÓS: Why an airplane?

HILLARY: Because you almost died in an airplane, and she is scared of jumping. And someday she'll have to jump. Furthermore, symbols are as real as what you think is ordinary realness.

MIKLÓS: Okay, then we go. [Mari laughs]

HILLARY: Wonderful. Because right now, he just showed you he is non-ordinary. It's a powerful thing for you two to bring home an airplane given what happened to you both.

We went on to discuss their life as if it were an ongoing movie and that they should live the next month with a more fascinating script, filled with surprises that would delight a future audience. Several weeks later, Miklós requested a session alone.

MIKLÓS: I truly liked the way you talked with me last session. It was so creative and clever at the same time. It really surprised and delighted me that you told us to think about our lives like a movie script. That brought something new to me. At first, I thought it didn't make sense to buy that toy, that it was just something silly. But then when you explained it to me I understood. I liked that very much. I also liked that you didn't try to pretend that I'm not dying. You didn't sugarcoat it and say to me, "Oh don't worry, you won't die." Because of that, I felt we could have a real conversation. I understand the point you made, that I should live every day like it is my last day, so each day has to be a special day. I have been thinking about this—that we are all dying or don't know when we might die, so we should live as fully as possible. This is having an impact on my decision about what I want to do with my health and whether I want to undergo treatment. I have not changed anything yet about how I am living. I'm still going to work and continue on as if everything was normal. The only thing we decided to do was take a spontaneous holiday, because the opportunity arose and we took it. This is probably in part because of what we talked about. Otherwise, I continue on as normal. I'm in a quite important project at work, which will last for a few weeks more. I think I would not like to just drop it. There are several people relying on me. This is where I am at the moment. I still have to face some difficult decisions about my health. I have many questions. I don't know how to talk about my feelings with my wife. Not because I can't talk about it—I think it would be a relief for me. But I worry about upsetting her. She wants to remain hopeful. She keeps telling me that I am better than I was a few weeks ago and that maybe this is a sign of recovery. But I know that this is only a temporary result due to the steroids I received. My condition is incurable. When she says this I just say, "okay" and agree with her, but I don't want to encourage her hopefulness. I know you don't know her well enough to judge enough how well she will be able to bare life without me, and I also know that you are not here to give me medical advice. I just feel that I need some help with how to handle talking to my wife. At this point I have the feeling that I am in a situation where I should make a decision about which way to go—whether I should continue treatment or not.

I know that you don't know any of my medical details and cannot discuss that aspect with me, but in general terms I don't really know how to make such a decision. These are my most immediate concerns.

BRAD: Of course no one knows what the best decision is for you regarding treatment. Even doctors will have different opinions. It is good for your clear mind to weigh all the facts and make the best decision that only you can make. But we can certainly talk about how to bring as much life as you can into every day that you have, and especially in ways that are gifts to your wife. In all the many years that you have been together, did you ever sing your wife a song?

MIKLÓS: No.

HILLARY: [Brad laughs] I thought that was the case. One wonderful surprise for her would be for you to sing her a song.

MIKLÓS: Well, she has heard me singing in the shower, for instance. [Miklós laughs] One time we were at the public baths and I was standing under a waterfall and it felt so good that somehow, I started singing and she heard me. The songs she has heard me singing are songs that people don't really hear in public. You probably don't know about them, but they are Communist songs. [Miklós laughs]

BRAD: This is what I think. Your wife is worried most about one thing—and it will be the same worry every day for the rest of your life. Every day she will worry whether you are happy. In spite of it all, she will wonder if you are happy. If every day for the rest of your life—for however long that is—she hears you sing, she'll say, "The last years of his life were the happiest, because I heard him sing. Even on the last day."

HILLARY: There can be no greater gift to her than her hearing you sing every day for the rest of your life.

MIKLÓS: [Smiles] I understand, but I think there is a difficulty. You can suggest this because you are full of songs, but I am not. I'm not a very musical type of person. I like songs, but I don't know many.

HILLARY: Which is why when she hears you singing, she will know that you must be truly happy.

MIKLÓS: I don't know many songs.

HILLARY: It doesn't matter.

BRAD: It would really surprise her if you once in a while learned a new song. She would be shocked. Leave some recordings for her. She can come home and find a note next to a recording that says, "Play." She'll play it and feel you. Every day she will be surprised by how she will receive a song. She might be taking a shower and then you sing outside the door. She might be fixing dinner and you sing, or you both might walk through the park and then you start singing. There are many ways. Maybe you decide to make a videotape of you singing. If you leave her a song every day, she will smile the rest of her life knowing that you had the happiest days and sang to the very last moment.

HILLARY: It's fine to give gifts, and it's fine to have short getaways together—that's wonderful and I know you're the kind of man that will do that and give her surprises. But nothing brings happiness to another person like hearing the sound of someone they love singing. Especially if you don't think you're a good singer. It's even more meaningful that way.

MIKLÓS: But I don't really feel happy these days. There are moments of course when I feel happy, but in general I don't feel happy. Is it okay to sing to her as if I am happy when I'm not?

BRAD: I can tell you an important lesson that comes from the history of America. The African slaves who lived in the south had the hardest lives. Their lives were unimaginably difficult and full of suffering. Yet the songs that came from those people during slavery times are some of the most important and beautiful songs in history. They didn't sing because they were happy. They sang because singing is what brought happiness. You don't have to be happy to sing.

HILLARY: In your case, you will sing to make her happy. It will make you happy when you see her happy. All the words you speak to her won't matter, because words are difficult. Words get caught up in logic and trying to make this point or that point, but music is about your heart having wings and lifting the emotions.

BRAD: This is what I think. I may be wrong, but I have never heard of a man in your situation who sang every day to his wife in as many ways as he could through the end of his life. You may be the first. So, you could devote the rest of your life to being a singer.

MIKLÓS: My worry is that I don't know how this illness will progress and if I will be forced to be in the hospital for a long period. If that is the case, she will come every day and have to see me just lying there, sick. Under those circumstances I can't promise you that I will be able to sing.

BRAD: You can tell her, "Please come here, I want to whisper something to you." Then you can whisper just a few musical bars. That's all it will take. Even in your last breath, you can sing a couple of measures. Now you should think about all the ways that song can come into your life that it perhaps won't be able to come into your life in the future.

HILLARY: For example, maybe you need tickets to the orchestra, maybe you need to upgrade your stereo, or buy more music. Now is the time to bring more music into your life. You might hire a band to come to your house - they could play while you sing a song. That would be extraordinary. [Miklós laughs]

Now is the time to give it everything you've got, doing everything you currently can do.

BRAD: And then the performance will change as time passes and you go through different stages. But all the words you can write, all the things anyone can say, and all the gifts you could give her, will not communicate to her as meaningfully and as authentically and as deeply that your reaching inside to sing her a song, in some way, every day. Music is the only language that conveys this sort of thing. She'll know it's for her because she'll know that you are trying to make her happy. This will make you happy. If you were going to learn some new songs, what songs would surprise her?

MIKLÓS: I like Gershwin very much. Maybe I should learn some of those songs.

BRAD: Ahhhh. Yes. Gershwin is so wonderful.

MIKLÓS: Those songs would be easy to learn and then she would feel what is inside me?

HILLARY: Do you know the Gershwin song, "Our Love is Here to Stay?"

MIKLÓS: Yes, it is wonderful.

BRAD: Do you know the story of that song?

MIKLÓS: I don't know the story.

HILLARY: As you know, George Gershwin wrote songs with his brother, Ira. At one point, George was diagnosed with an inoperable brain tumor. Many people assume that that song is just a romantic love song. What many people don't realize is that George Gershwin wrote that song for his brother. It is a song from one brother to another who both know they will be parted by death. It is one of our favorite songs.

[Brad gets up and walks over to his piano and then sings to Miklós]

BRAD: Listen to what a difference music makes [then he sings]:

All you have to do
is put on the music
it changes the room
no matter what kind of trouble you have
it brings a joy
and when George was dying, he just said to his brother ...

[Brad now begins the song "Our Love is Here to Stay," playing it slowly. Hillary and Brad sing the words]

Oh my dear,
our love is here to stay
together we're
going a long, long way
In time the Rockies may crumble
Gibraltar may tumble
we're only made of clay
Our love is here
to stay

[Brad brings the song to a close. Miklós is smiling widely]

BRAD: I'm so happy that you like George Gershwin. When I was a little boy and everyone else wanted to a baseball player or a doctor or in the movies, I just wanted to be George Gershwin. [Brad begins to play "Embraceable You" and he sings Miklós the following altered lyrics to its melody:]

Your wife is going to be so happy
to hear you sing
Nothing could be sweeter
all the money all the gifts
nothing could be finer
than you singing a Gershwin song
What else can convey
the love
you have for her?
A Gershwin song
is inside the heart of everyone
You know that
you didn't hesitate to know
that you wanted George Gershwin songs

[Brad brings the song to a close]

BRAD: So, which one Gershwin song will be the first one?

MIKLÓS: [Smiles] I don't know. Maybe the song, "Summertime."

[Brad continues to play another Gershwin melody]

BRAD: Do you have a piano?

MIKLÓS: No.

HILLARY: You could always rent a piano and have someone come over to back you up. [Miklós laughs] That would be something special. She would never forget that. [Brad brings the music to a close]

BRAD: You didn't know we would be talking about George Gershwin today, did you? Even on a foggy day, there's a Gershwin song in the air. [Brad laughs] You've got to strike up the band. Because somewhere, in your home, someone needs you to watch over her. [Brad and Miklós laugh]

HILLARY: If you sing like that, your love is going to be here to stay. We just need to know: Are you going to sing your wife some Gershwin songs? Will you sing about the "way she looks tonight?"

MIKLÓS: Yes, I will do it. I really like these songs, so I can do it. I wouldn't perform them for an audience, but for her I can do this.

BRAD: Wonderful. What an interesting Broadway show is about to come inside your home: Music from the Communist Party and George Gershwin! [Everyone laughs] The marquee will read, "From the Kremlin to Tin Pan Alley." [Everyone laughs. There is a long pause]

HILLARY: We, of course, could come up with many more things for you to do. Including sometimes you should perform in costume, or hire an accompaniment. That would really blow her mind. There is no end to what you can do. A man like you should go all the way or least consider performing everything.

BRAD: I'm going to paint a picture of something you probably won't do, but if you did it, it would probably be the greatest moment in her life. Hire a whole company—a choir and orchestra to come into your house. Perform three Gershwin songs with you singing on the microphone. Or rent a concert hall and take her there and say, "This show is for you." Even if it's only one song, that would be unbelievable.

MIKLÓS: That would be something very strange for me and to her as well. We are not into big productions.

BRAD: I think you should experiment with any size production including a home cabaret. If you shoot for one song a day, you might be surprised at what you come up with. I just know, no matter how it's done, whether it's a cappella, with a record, or a band, that you will be showing her that you are considering every possible way to express your heart with song and to give her this gift every day.

HILLARY: This is the greatest gift you can give her. The main question for you is, "On what stage will you perform the rest of your life?" I think a musical stage is one of the best ways to show the one you love, what is in your heart. There will be competing stages—some will say that you should be on the medical stage. But you can say, "Nah, this is show business. I'm on a musical stage. Even if I'm in a hospital bed."

BRAD: No matter what song you sing, no matter how you sing it, or what the words are, it always brings the ultimate message, "I'm happy

> because our love is here to stay." That song was written when George was in his final days. There will be a lot of talk between you and your wife coming up. But past all the talk, your singing voice needs to rise above it all, telling her, "Our love makes me happy every day." That is the greatest gift. This is the time for love to be triumphant, to have the ultimate final say.

Why not make your creative therapy life a musical? Do you prefer a Gershwin tune or are you more inclined to invite a Stephen Sondheim song? Every kind of music has been performed on the Broadway, London, Paris, and Budapest stages, so feel free to produce whatever touches and lifts your heart. Find the songs that deliver the pulse of life and musically celebrate the change that can forever stay. Set up the scenery and props for a magnificent finale, doing so every day as if it's the last day of your life. Procure costumes, makeup, and whatever you want that makes it a life-changing and death-changing cabaret.

Be ready to break into a song, whether it is sung loudly or through a faint whisper. We invite you to replace your alarm clock with a musical overture to announce the beginning of each creative therapy day. Even consider hanging a theater curtain in your living room. Or draw one on the wall, no matter how large or small. We used to have a red velvet theater curtain in our living room and now have a painting of a curtain that opens to reveal a green chile pepper. Put up any kind of curtain rather than a peekaboo glass and remind yourself that your life can step onto the musical stage.

Ask John Cage what it means to escape the therapy cage: "Everything we do is music." Place a sign somewhere that names the musical you are in. Perhaps it simply says, *Bob: The Musical* or *Suzie and the Dreamgirls*, or bring back your revival of *My Fair Lady*, *Oklahoma*, *The Sound of Music*, *Camelot*, *Spamelot*, *110 in the Shade*, *Merrily We Roll Along*, *Company*, *Godspell*, *Jesus Christ Superstar*, *Ain't Misbehavin'*, *Annie*, *Les Misérables*, *Mary Poppins*, *Fiddler on the Roof*, *West Side Story*, *The Music Man*, *The King and I*, *The Producers*, *Hello, Dolly*, *Porgy and Bess*, *A Chorus Line*, *Finian's Rainbow*, *Gigi*, *Peter Pan*, *The Lion King*, *Fame*, *Show Boat*, *Matilda*, *The Book of Mormon*, *Pippin*, *Wicked*, or *Carousel*, to mention a few of the long list of hit shows.

Surprise yourself and others with more creative dialogue, singing interludes, dance routines, and comedic relief. Install a spotlight if you wish or at least bring out a flashlight that can spot more action. Stop all modeled and muddled therapy. It's too much a chore and bore when you can take the stage and make life more real by making it more unreal. Bring the lighting, sound, movement, and creative lines that deliver the reprise of ongoing surprise. Stop sitting in the audience and quit milling about backstage. You are already over-rehearsed. You know how to communicate and act even when you try to appear that you are not communicating and not acting. The theater of creative therapy waits to host your performance.

If it's a good day to live, then it's a good day to die. It's an even better time for the premiere of your musical performance. Prepare for the dramatic changes of your life. You only need a heart that longs for a song. After the Rockies crumble and Gibraltar tumbles, we turn back to clay and dust. Even after all the days of youth and age are done, after the whole pie is gone, after the many feathers have blown away, after all the Kofola and champagne are poured, after the violins and songs are put away, and after the fairy tale pretends to end, you can still celebrate that love, wonder, joy, and change are here to stay.

PART III
Epilogue

"Life is a lot like jazz … it's best when you improvise."

George Gershwin

13

CREATIVE THERAPY IS JAZZ

When asked about the nature of jazz performance, Louis Armstrong replied, "What we play is life." Creative therapy is experiential jazz that plays the whole spectrum of human expression—its creative changes help improvise a new life. Since we never know what a client will communicate, surprise is assured and welcomed. No matter what a client brings to a session—whether it is a rock, a raccoon, a straw, a ghost, an owl, a sketchpad, tap dance shoes, or a piano—jam with it. Masterful improvisation is what carries a session forward. Improvise, embellish, and alter in order to create a fresh performance filled with unexpected changes that can even make a worn-out routine or over-played conversation loop come aesthetically alive. As jazz saxophonist John Coltrane wonderfully rephrased this latter point, "You can play a shoestring if you're sincere." The creative therapist sincerely wants to alchemically turn heavy verbal lead into uplifting experiential gold, knowing that interspersed creative action rather than uninterrupted narration is required.

The Art of Making Art Out of Error: It All Starts with Creative Technique

Without mastery of technique, neither musician nor therapist has the skills or chops to perform. Even improvisation must be practiced and learned. The legendary prodigious pianist Art Tatum said it bluntly: "You have to practice improvisation, let no one kid you about it!" This is not to imply that you need to become perfect, always saying the right thing or unfailingly exhibiting the correct action. What you must master is the art of utilizing (making practical and effective use of) whatever is presented in the moment.

When we train budding creative therapists, we approach it as a performing art and offer creative therapeutic technique, emphasizing practice and performance over theory and explanation (see H. Keeney & B. Keeney, 2013). In particular, we teach them to not carelessly dismiss a mistake and overlook its potential contribution to the ongoing action. We show them how to instead immediately incorporate it in an unexpected, resourceful manner. The creativity of creative therapy can be most alive when a presumed error or failure is brilliantly turned to reveal a difference that leads to change or shows the hidden sign of a previously unnoticed success.

Error helps make the performance right. As the idiosyncratic pianist Thelonious Monk advised, perform so that "wrong is right." Creative therapy experiments with difference and this especially includes working with the errors and deviations that are the right kind of wrongs that lead to the promised land of unexpected invention. Tenor saxophonist Coleman Hawkins, sometimes called "Hawk" or "Bean," expressed the need for this same kind of mistake-seeking performance: "If you don't make mistakes, you aren't really trying." The creative therapist immediately offers an invitation to change, paradoxically doing so to better assure that it will bring a living mistake rather than a dead "right" into the room. Without this kind of difference, there is no way to make a real difference.

Even if a client reports, "I'm worse now," you can quietly think to yourself or celebrate out loud with your client: "Excellent, we learned how it is possible for you to change!" Any kind of difference is an excellent learning outcome that can be used to invent other actions aimed in more resourceful directions. For instance, if a client learns to gain exactly one pound of weight, no more and no less, then a skill involving *weight control* has been acquired that can subsequently steer the body elsewhere. This might begin with instruction to hang out near a kitchen cabinet that is arranged to have one pound less food content in its space than it did before. Or the client can be sent to explore the section of a bookstore where the reading material is lighter. Perhaps it is foolishly wise to bring a small food scale to measure the books to assure the purchase is exactly one pound. For a client who chronically worries about how long the next panic attack will last, help him learn to shorten the amount of time spent reading the news or make sure that however long he worries, he agrees to spend twice that time sharpening pencils. Why? Only ask that question afterwards, making sure to dwell on it for an agreed upon duration of time in a different part of the session room, while demonstrating how you sharpen a pencil or keep some meaningless, non-troublesome books on your shelf. Experiments in altering time and space can be applied to any activity including their design during a brief walk around the most fascinating part of a park where you reflect on the value of misinterpreting the assignment. Restage your errors so they are invitations to make some jazz.

Creative therapists utilize rather than demonize errors in others, themselves, their surroundings, and especially the real-time interactions taking place in a session. As musician Brian Eno said, "honor thy error" as the guide to creating a change. This is the pragmatic start-up for cybernetic action—an error offers a difference that can be reoriented to help turn a virtuous wheel of change. Jazz improvisation and creative therapy are examples of embodied cybernetics, the art of making art out of error. Here an error is better reconceived as a "difference," "diferencia," "differenza," "unterscheid," "különbség," "diferença," "разница," "区别," "差," or "umehluko, that helps improvise the next action that keeps the performance different than expected.

We once had a supervisee who was surprised to hear us celebrate "first-order cybernetics" and mentioned she had read a book in graduate school that claimed that it was "bad" for therapy. Her professor had explained that all ideas associated with it should be avoided because it might turn a therapist into an engineer who no longer wants to hear a conversation, choosing instead to treat a client system as if it was a "black box" or a "machine." We chose not to get into an interpretive debate that pointed out that therapy texts are often plagued with shoddy scholarship and misinformation. In addition, we chose not to obliquely say: "Would you believe an author who similarly advises therapists to avoid studying 'linguistics' because it makes you treat people like dictionaries?" Instead, we responded more directly: "Yes, some theories are scolded, spanked, ostracized, and banned by those unable to recognize the unique gift and resourceful difference they bring if greeted with a virtuous circular interaction. We personally welcome cybernetics to our New Orleans home, and this especially includes all its error-prone ways. In the room of improvisation, there is no need to quarrel about interpretation. There you invite the playfulness of jazz and discover that cybernetics really knows how to change and cook a tune and a session. The cybernetics you heard about in graduate school tragically went into the wrong room where it was given a life sentence in a book rather than taken to Mardi Gras or the Jazz Festival. Come and introduce yourself to our ragtime, stride, and bebop cybernetics who is always our muse and friend. The way she performs can help you have a great jam session."

A creative therapist, like a jazz performer, learns that it is wiser and more gracious to commune with errors rather than excommunicate them from the conversation because it helps lead to a fruitful outcome. As Art Tatum said: "There is no such thing as a wrong note." Don't emphasize the adjective "wrong" because it ends enjoyment of the song. Choose to accentuate the "note" without any prior or post interpretation so the only concern is what note to perform next, enabling the tune to generatively keep going. Creative therapy makes itself optimally ready to utilize the notes that are typically considered a blooper, goof, mistake, or pratfall. They are not interpreted as indications of what is wrong with the client, family, or culture; they are regarded as bringing an opportunity for creative improvisation. Reach for the difference and avoid the negative interpretive connotation that misses the gift. The "error" that is practically connoted by cybernetics is the jazz musician's and creative therapist's valued "note." Go ahead and jam with rather than damn what differs.

Play What's Not There

The jazz of creative therapy heeds the advice of the milestone trumpet master, Miles Davis: "Don't play what's there, play what's not there." In other words, become skilled at inventing and interspersing that which is uncommon, as well as discerning what ought to remain unspoken. This is no easy task for a beginning performer, whether on the therapy or music stage. Bebop trumpeter Dizzy Gillespie reminds us: "It's taken me all my life to learn what not to play." The creative therapist may have to work just as hard to *not* play the standard lines and well-known techniques of therapy models as they do to invent original action in the moment—learning what *not* to say as well as inventing a new line.

We had a client who made her living as a therapist. Though she said she was depressed, we couldn't help but notice that she had an unusual nervous habit. Before saying anything to her children she would robotically ask their permission to talk: "May I say something?" Though it was probably meant to be a ritual-like genuflection of respect, it was an obvious irritant to her family. Her children even mocked her with the family pet. "Celeste, do we have your permission to offer you a treat?" She confessed that this habit had become like a "tic" and that it started several years ago during her therapy training. Furthermore, this same repeating question was the most commonly spoken phrase in each of her sessions. She and her family wanted the robotic tic to end, bringing back a real mom with more natural talk.

We proceeded to act: "Are you here because you'd like us to share what we recommend?" After confirming she had come to receive our help, we continued: "Thank you. Now we don't need to ask you that question again or whether it's okay for us to speak, because we all agree why we're here. Remember that whatever we say or do from this moment on will be different than everyday talk and etiquette. We are here to help you experience a change that will make a difference in the way your life sounds. Your change might be found in something else that is said or discovered in what is no longer said. There was a jazz musician who once claimed that it took most of his life to figure out what not to play. You're ahead of him, because you already know what you don't want to say. One more thing, you should leave now and go purchase a hand cricket, that little pocket toy that makes the sound of a cricket when you press it. Your children can help you find it either online or at a toy store. Whenever you feel that tic wanting to click in the next session, click the clicker instead. Make that verbal tic a handheld click. And one more thing, everyone in the family needs to have their own clicker. This family needs more click and less tic. Now go home and sound like the crickets are alive."

Jamming with Interpretation

The creative therapist is freer to use any kind of interpretation in any kind of manner rather than fixate on advocating a previously chosen one. Even a random metaphor can be creatively woven into an evocative, change-inducing theme as long as it expands the room and inspires the therapist to keep the session moving toward change rather than drift into pontification. The bummer brought by canned or overly theoretical interpretation is that it only assures that a session will feel boring and creatively dead. In addition, the therapist becomes dissociated from the ongoing action and far removed from a fresh source of inspiration.

The creative therapist creatively invents and constantly changes contextual themes that are comparable to music's harmony, giving underlying dissonance and consonance to the ongoing action line that is more like music's melodic line. As important are the dramatic tropes or "twists and turns" that change the performance climate by specifying different ways of regarding a conversational theme. These include allegory, hyperbole, irony, metaphor, metonymy (association by proximity), antanaclasis (having fun with pun), oxymoron (ostensible self-contradiction), and synecdoche (part-whole inversions). Here we find that most therapists advance the same kind of trope—allegory (interpretation of hidden meanings) and it rarely has fun with pun. Therapy as a textual *and* dramatic form is far too literal, critical, allegorically metaphorical, and overly serious, locked into unchanging forms of expression than is necessary. Emotionless expression, passionless tone, frozen body movement, zero creative energy, and an overly serious countenance do not make a moving performance. The presence of shifting tropes is a better sign that a session has come to life. With action embellishment and freshly invented themes, therapy jazz arrives to save the session from missing a beat and losing its song.

In creative therapy, stuck situations are characterized by overly redundant spoken lines and uninspired action in need of change. Sometimes a session benefits from more cacophony, dissonance, consonance, resolution, simplicity, complexity, chaos, order, nonsense, or clarity. When such a change is made, it is analogous to the recovery and resurrection of a boring tune made well by creative invention that doctors the trite performance convention. Dr. John and Professor Longhair stand ready to make a house call for any performance blues. In therapy, the client's reality is in need of some aesthetic excitement rather than a dampening of spirit or the killing of soulful possibility. In other words, less tic and more click. Turn a session upside down, pull it inside out, or jump to another track to help change break out. Doctor the whole performance journey to make it more attractive to change. Nothing less can bring a session back to life.

Don't talk about your sessions; enact a change. As Thelonious Monk said of jazz, "Talking about music is like dancing about architecture." Talking about therapy is the same. Make sure to get the word strings and the theoretical cobwebs out of your head when you perform with a client. Remember what Paul Desmond, the great saxophonist replied when asked what he thought about when he played on stage: "I think I had it in the back of my mind that I wanted to sound like a dry martini." You are better off thinking about baking a chocolate cake or throwing out a fishing line than getting lost in a tower of babble.

We worked with a family constellations therapist who said his life lacked fulfillment and excitement. He felt out of tune and out of sync with his work, feeling he had made the wrong career choice. Saying he wanted to retool his life, he regretted he had not pursued science like he had wanted to when he was a boy. Brad, who won the international science fair in 1969, asked him if he ever had a science project in his youth. He lit up and said, "Yes! And that was the happiest time of my life." He described how he had collected water samples from local ponds and studied the pollution caused by a nearby factory. We asked, "Did you ever build a telescope?" He replied, "I'm amazed you asked me that. I could never afford to buy the one I wanted but owning a telescope was my childhood dream. My parents always felt sorry they were not able to give me this gift." In an instant we knew where the session would go because it doesn't take a rocket scientist to see the metaphorical link between two kinds of constellations. We proceeded to get his pledge to finish unfinished business in his family of origin—fulfilling the dream of his childhood. We discussed whether he'd buy a telescope kit and assemble it or buy all the parts separately. In addition, we asked if he'd be happier grinding his own lenses or buying ones already made. Of course, we had to ask whether his telescope would be a reflector or a refractor. At the end we offered another prescription: "Every night before going to sleep, close your eyes and imagine looking at a clear night sky with stars twinkling everywhere. There you are in the middle of this scene with a telescope in hand or carefully placed on a stand. There is a family around you waiting their turn to see and discuss the sky. Then you realize you are no longer sure whether you've become an astronomer who wonders about the stars or a therapist who constellates rather than procrastinates completing unfinished business. Even more shocking is that you don't care anymore because with a telescope underneath the sky, you feel you found your place in the universe."

Rhythm: Bringing It All to Life

Even with good action lines and colorful thematic accompaniment, it takes vibrant rhythm to bring it all together and make the jazz of creative therapy come alive. Therapists and clients can say all the right things and explore endless intriguing themes, but if the session isn't carried on a buoyant rhythm, it will sink. The aliveness, soul, and flow of a session come from what stride pianist Fats Waller said about rhythm: "You get that right tickin' rhythm, man, and it's ON!" The great jazz composer Duke Ellington went on to further accentuate this meaning: "It don't mean a thing if it ain't got that swing." Perhaps he later added, "It don't mean it swings if it ain't got that tingling thing."

The creative therapist knows that a session must rock and sway on each fulcrum of change until it tips forward into the next act and operation. Such movement isn't contemplated; it is enacted and expressed through rhythm and tempo. The therapist's body must be in the room, not just the talking and reflecting head. When a session rhythmically swings like jazz, whether the tempo is fast or slow, it feels alive with soul. This swing is both felt and expressed by the therapist's body through rocking, swaying, and a non-monotonous rhythm in speech. When a soulful rhythm is cooking, the client will also catch it and the session will wake up. Catching, creating, sustaining, or changing rhythm is rarely, if ever, discussed in psychotherapy education. Instead, therapy is exemplified by boring, soulless, and rhythm-less conversation. It's time to bring on the jazz and go for the somatic tingle and creative sizzle. Here is a secret that will change the way you do therapy: Before every session, turn on your inner jukebox and catch a rhythm—any rhythm is fine, but the livelier and more soulful, the better. Hear that rhythm inside you as you rock, sway, and bounce your body until you feel the beat take hold. Your movements don't have to be large or pronounced, although it's fine if they are; let your body lead the way. When it's time to start your session, keep this inner rhythm going in the background, circulating like a current or pulse that is more prominent than your overly conscious mind. You may appear relatively still on the outside, but your unconscious will be jamming on the inside, awake and ready to participate. It's simply too difficult to make a session creatively come to life when your whole body and unconscious are comatose. Artist Henri Matisse once said, "Jazz is rhythm and meaning." So is therapy, but the rhythm has been forgotten, though it's one of the greatest resources available to therapists who want to make their sessions creatively cook.

Here the equivalent of a melodic line, harmonic circle, and rhythmic swing must all come together to make a session cook. It must have a heartbeat, the ecstatic pulse that enables transformative change to be felt and brought home. After Hurricane Katrina hit New Orleans, we saw a court-ordered case with a family that had lost their home in the Lower Ninth Ward and had to move to a FEMA trailer outside the city. The boy had suddenly started angrily beating on walls, causing physical damage wherever he went—especially at home and school. Without missing a beat, we said: "We know that the Lower Ninth Ward is full of musical families, and each family tends to carry on one particular instrument. Some families pass on the horn, and others make sure it's the clarinet, tuba, or drum that marches on with each generation. Which instrument is it for your family?" The mother immediately answered, "We are a proud family of drummers." To the surprise of the family, we immediately responded, "There's no more need to find out what's going on here. Your son needs a pair of drumsticks, so he can better practice his rhythm and experiment with a quick tempo rather than a quick temper. A boy like this with a destiny and a calling to drum will find that it's more satisfying to beat a drum skin with drumsticks than bang on a wall or kick a trashcan." The boy and his family became excited and felt freed to be more creatively interesting and better aesthetically prepared to continue the musical tradition that had been interrupted by an unexpected storm. The rest of the session discussed all the different kinds of drumsticks waiting to be purchased at the music store. We insisted on contributing a pair as our gift, honoring the musicians who make New Orleans sound better than other places in the world. We gave them some cash and sent them on their way to the music store, a more suitable place than a mental health clinic to find a better way to get the right beat. We wished we had remembered to tell them that Miles Davis used to say: "My ego only needs a good rhythm section." We would have restated it with the family's choice of metaphor: "My temper only needs a good rhythm section."

There Are Two Kinds of Sessions

Duke Ellington famously said: "There are two kinds of music. Good music, and the other kind." The same is true for therapy. A session either cooks or it doesn't cook. All the elaborate talk and theory in the world cannot hide the experiential fact that some sessions are dead as a mackerel and should be questioned as to why they got any air time. Like jazz, therapy should prioritize great performances rather than obsessing over which models and theories are being used. After all, improvisation is done in the moment; there isn't time to ruminate before playing the next note. Miles Davis summarized this in one eloquent sentence: "I'll play it first and tell you what it is afterwards." First, evaluate whether a school of therapy offers inspiring creative sessions and then don't bother to check out its theory if it doesn't. This action alone is enough to revolutionize the profession.

Often a creative therapist, like a jazz musician, must first get lost and then accidentally found in order to good music. Thelonious Monk makes this point quite dramatically: "Where's jazz going? I don't know? Maybe it's going to hell. You can't make anything go anywhere. It just happens." A session surely goes to hell and does not come back if a therapist focuses on what existentially narrows and chills. The only way out of this hell-bound shrinkage is to blow the horn, play the drum, change the musical key, tune the string, strike the gong, or whatever it takes to send in the brass, wind, and percussion of change. Only the enacted performance of change, no matter its metaphorical instrument, can call forth the change of atmosphere that is more conducive to bringing out the jazz of life.

As a young man, Brad had a colleague who seemed hell-bent on proving that she was a *bona fide* hypochondriac. She confided in him, mentioning her involvement with nearly a dozen doctors who treated ailments that never seemed to end and while questioning whether they had ever begun. At the heart of her suffering was a growing anxiety about being unable to produce any dramatic change in a session. She didn't deny it—she was worried about her inability to do good therapy like those she had formerly studied and admired. Everyone in the clinical workplace doubted whether she had enough chops to enter the room with a client. It was no wonder that she had spine issues, dermatological rashes, gastrointestinal pain, insomnia, laryngitis, restless leg syndrome, and other kinds of symptoms. She felt she needed to talk to someone so Brad compassionately listened.

To this day, Brad still regrets only listening to her and providing emotional support, but not offering the kind of prescription we now offer. If we could return to that moment in time we would say something like: "It sounds like your life is hell—that's the word you chose to describe it. Maybe you should make hell more interesting, so you could at least have a few minutes of enjoyment. Instead of going behind the one-way mirror so often when you aren't sure what to do in a session, why not wear a paper sack over your head with holes for your eyes, nose, and mouth. [At that time there was a well-known comic named "The Unknown Comic" who performed with a paper sack over his head.] The next time you leave the room, tell the family that you are going to invite "The Unknown Therapist" to come in the room and offer some advice. Then leave the room, put on your paper bag, and return ready to be different. There's nothing like a mask to change the actor and the performance. What do you have to lose? Why not visit a costume shop rather than see another doctor? Wear a mask and don't ask why. Just do it to unmask another way of being in the room."

Later, we found traditional healing traditions in which masks are regularly worn by the healer while other masks worn by the client. This enabled them to step onto a bigger existential stage and different reality where they could more dramatically enact healing. Whether the mask a creative therapist wears is visible or invisible, change it if the performance role needs a costume change or a change in role. In other words, unmask the creative therapist in every session. Years after Brad left New York City, he couldn't resist the urge to wear a paper sack over his head in a family therapy session in Texas. The young boy in the family got excited and demanded his own sack. Instantly Brad had a connection with the boy and the family that wasn't there before. The moral of this true story is this: when a session is going nowhere and needs to be sacked, wear a sack. Or go already prepared and wear socks that don't match—one green and the other red in case a client asks what that is about. You'll then be ready to say: "One sock says 'stop' and the other says 'go.'"

Studying Master Performances

It's important to study previously performed creative therapy sessions. Examining these classic renditions provides access to more detail about what improvised changes made a difference in how the session moved. John Coltrane remarked: "I've found you've got to look back at the old things and see them in a new light." As you learn to see creative therapy under the new light of jazz, more and different dynamics will stand out revealing the underlying circularity of it all. Creative action evokes new creative understanding, which in turn, breeds another unexpected action. Each new change leads to the next level of change. This is well articulated by saxophone colossus Sonny Rollins: "This is my dilemma: I'm a guy who makes things up as I go along so nothing is ever finished—there are so many layers. So, when you solo, yeah, you might get into one thing, but then, hey, everything has implications! You can hear the next level. And that's how I feel about improvising—there's always another level."

We sometimes instruct trainees to read a published therapy transcript and stop midway through. Then they are asked to improvise the rest of the session, writing out what they would say next, how the client would respond, and so on. After this is done, they go back and see what the other therapist actually did. Trainees then learn that every different action has its immediate implications and there is never just one way to improvise a session. The creative therapist is always searching for how to create better lines and therapeutic moves than what was previously performed. This helps the therapist keep growing and changing so that learning is never finished. For therapy to be more change-filled, the therapist must become more willing, able, and ready to change the way they improvise the twists and turns of each freshly composed performance.

Evolving Your Own Style

There is also a lot to be learned from studying how other improvisational performers from any professional guild learned how to evolve a unique style of expression. Most great masters developed their own style by first imitating a master. We not only instruct students to study the transcriptions of masterful therapy, but we also recommend they pick a favorite session, memorize it, and learn to perform it exactly like the therapist—complete with accent, vocal intonation, and body language. This dramatic enactment helps develops performance skill, but it also gets students to pay more attention to the unique style of great therapists, expanding their sense of what is possible in therapeutic expression.

While imitation of master performers is a vital part of development, eventually there comes a time for every performer, whether a jazz musician or creative therapist, to make the big creative leap into their own style, drawing more upon what is unique about their own personal, relational, and situational resources. This creative leap must come at the right time and should not be pushed prematurely, however. First, you need a good launch pad—the chops to play like the masters—before the countdown to blast off can begin.

Once the creative ascent is made, everything about you becomes inseparable from improvised change—you are jazz. Only then will you both know and feel who you are and what you previously were trying to become. As Heinz von Foerster once quipped, "To know yourself, change." Only through changing how you perform can you discover what you're made of. The pioneer of cool jazz, Chet Baker, advised: "Well, if I could play like Wynton (Marsalis), I wouldn't play like Wynton." Multi-instrumentalist Roland Kirk further reminds us that after each session, we must return again to find ourselves still searching for how we can bring forth the change that never remains the same for long, the mystery of changing the way things change: "So until we see you again, bright moments and keep searchin' for your mystery note on the universal piano of life."

If needed, wear a purple bolo tie that resembles an Ericksonian costume induction. When it's time for the big leap, add another color to make your life more than the color purple. Why not wear the circular earrings of Virginia Satir in order to better hear and sculpt the circularity of a family system? Or adopt a foreign accent that sounds like Salvador Minuchin, but then alter it slightly so it sounds unique to you. We supervised a therapy graduate student who struggled to speak clearly and articulately in her sessions. Though she spoke naturally and fluently outside of therapy, as soon as she was with clients she stumbled on her words. It made her feel and appear nervous and inept, which led her to ask for help. That night Brad had a dream that he told the student to speak in a foreign accent with her clients. The next day Brad told the student about his dream. Being someone who was interested in dreams and creative imagination, she was at once inspired, intrigued, and petrified at the thought of speaking to clients in a foreign accent. She asked, "What kind of foreign accent?" Brad replied, "Well, since you like the therapy of Salvador Minuchin, why not speak with an Argentinian accent and throw in a few unexpected Spanish words since Minuchin was from Argentina."

The student agreed that was a good choice and recalled that she actually used to try speaking in foreign accents when she was younger to entertain her family. After practicing for a while with Hillary as they both tried to do their best Minuchin (which resulted in a lot of laughter), the student agreed to give the accent a try in her next session, despite now being more nervous than ever about how she would sound to the clients. Not only did the therapist smoothly conduct a whole session with an Argentinian accent, she learned the popular phrase "ponerse las pilas," which literally translates as "to put your batteries in." She went on to try out other accents with different clients. Sometimes she spoke without an accent but experimented with different ways of changing her pitch and cadence. The student not only stopped stumbling over her words, she developed her own conversational and performance style that helped launch her therapy to the next level. The lesson is that sometimes in order to get more of your natural gifts and originality coming through, you first have to perform like someone else, even stepping into the voice of someone you admire.

The Essence of a Great Creative Therapist

Saxophonist and bossa nova ambassador Stan Getz proposed that the four qualities essential to a great jazz performer are "taste, courage, individuality, and irreverence." These also pertain to a great creative therapist. Even when redundancy and stylistic habits appear in therapeutic work, each moment is approached in some kind of original way. Should you speak a line you have used before in another session, it will be performed differently rather than be a rehash if spoken at the right moment. Jazz original Ornette Coleman offered the same performance note: "Jazz is the only music in which the same note can be played night after night but differently each time."

We previously published a transcription of a session Brad conducted with a psychiatrist he saw in front of a live audience in Toronto (Keeney, 2011). The doctor began by lamenting that his sessions had gone dead and he seriously needed a creative boost. Brad asked, "What is the most boring thing you do in sessions?" The doctor replied, "I am sick and tired of asking a client how they feel about things." Brad then asked him to perform that lifeless line the way he habitually does it with clients: "How do you feel about that?" The rest of the session explored endless other ways of asking the same question that included giving it an Italian accent and dropping the other letters in "feel" and only saying "f." The newborn therapist found that "f" led to other words from "fear" to "failure" to "forgive," including a childhood fear of "flunking" school and a "forgotten" issue with his "father." None of these remarks were interpreted or conversationally explored; they were used as "fodder" to change the performance of all "f" words. His final prescription was to make himself a "fictionary" of "f" words. But before his project began,

Brad told him he first needed to get a new business card with a changed name: "Dr. F." He had that card made that very afternoon, and for nearly a decade he has sent us periodic progress reports that contain other creative embellishments of "f" words, always singing off with "Dr. F."

The Joint Is Jumpin'

There comes a time in the life of every performance artist, and this includes the creative therapist, when they are ready for bebop inventor Charlie Parker's ultimate recommendation: "Master your instrument, master the music, and then forget all that shit and just play." This advice came from someone who practiced music day and night. Beginning therapists must discipline themselves to get some therapeutic chops while at the same time study how others with more advanced learning have gone past theory and technique to become more open vessels for unimpeded improvisation.

The paradoxical situation is that the creative performer must begin trying to master that which must be later abandoned. Though this wisdom is often repeated as a platitude among therapists, it is rarely ever practiced. At the beginning of training, the aspirant looks to what lies ahead and inspirationally admires rather than indulges any jealous feelings about the mastery of the greats. When mastery of one's own style is finally attained, the big circle of change turns again as it is now time to turn around and take a look from behind. This is when the performer must re-acquire the beginner's mind necessary to bring back and create new ways of working with whatever valuable was thrown away. A common mistake and performance tragedy found among some therapy students and teachers is thinking that the abandonment of mastery should be done right away before there is anything to throw away. You can't "not know" in the Zen-like and master-like wisdom way until you first own some deeply engrained know-how. Too many therapists have conflated the "not knowing" of a master with the "not knowing what to do" of a beginner. You do not literally throw away any hard-earned chops (or the idea that you need to first learn them), you throw them out of your conscious mind into the deeper unconscious where they are better guided and regulated.

Finally, after enough years of practice that periodically acquires and retires this and that technique, pedagogical strategy, and higher learning, the fully cooked performer eventually comes to the place where the most important action is to make the hook up to the raw and primal creative life force and let it rip. Here the creative therapist becomes more like a traditional healer with no need to follow any model or get lost in debates over this way or that way, preferring to travel the mainline highway to change. Even practice as it was formerly known comes to an end as every moment becomes an invitation for an opening night performance. As the jazz legend Wes Montgomery referred to this final stage of development: "I never practice my guitar ... from time to time I just open the case and throw in a piece of raw meat."

The creative therapist is also ready to open a clinical case and throw in a piece of raw change. In one well-known creative therapy case, a young man in a Louisiana prison was advised to envision his bed as a boat and draw an alligator underneath it. He was further instructed to go to sleep at night with the goal of taking a dream adventure outside the prison walls. He subsequently not only dreamed of an outside swamp, he met a man who taught him how to carry a light and be safe around 'gators. We later gave him a passport to travel all over the world where he would find other gifts and valuable teachings waiting for him. Throwing this alligator meat in his life cut his prison sentence in half. "The Light Man," as this client called himself after a few sessions, was only there in the daytime and gone at night.

In another case, a family came with an eight-year-old son who constantly worried, believing he would soon die. He thought he had some kind of heart trouble, so the parents took him to a doctor, but nothing physically wrong was found. He still insisted that his days were numbered. During the session he drew a picture of an airplane and explained that his dad traveled a lot and that he also worried his plane might crash. Finally, he had been made upset at school because someone had told him that Santa Claus was not real. He assumed he would not live long enough for another holiday season and Christmas was about a month away.

The family was asked to designate one corner of their garage as an imaginary world. "Draw a circle on the floor; it has to be exactly two feet in diameter. This circle represents your new family world. Draw an ocean inside the circle and paint it blue. Use enamel paint so it won't easily fade. Sketch some landmasses in the circle as well and paint those green and brown, as it suits your world. When this is done, gather some small toy boats and place them on the sea. Identify one of those ships as your favorite. This shall be the family pirate ship. Make sure that you create your own pirate flag. There must also be secret names that you use with each other. These are to be your pirate names. When this work is all done, we want you to take turns making up stories about your adventures as a family of pirates. Together you will negotiate troubled waters and stormy seas. You will make great discoveries and celebrate victories in faraway places."

A week later the family sent a picture the boy had drawn as their flag. It was a ship with two masts in the middle. What was intriguing was how he depicted the ship balanced on three swords that were directly underneath it. These three swords held up the family ship. For several years, postcards were exchanged. Brief reports from the boy would mention exciting adventures at sea as postcards were sent to the family from all over the world. The last card received came about six years later. It was a picture of an old shipyard.

Soon after this, the father called saying that all had gone very well for all these years, but now the boy had started a troubling compulsive behavior. Every night he conducted a ritual where he faced every direction and made strange arm movements and hand gestures. What had begun as a one-minute brief sequence later escalated into a two-hour ordeal. The parents were afraid to see a local psychiatrist as friends and colleagues had advised. Brad agreed to have monthly phone calls with the boy instead of exchanging postcards. He first advised him to concentrate his ritual by making it last no longer than 30 seconds, assuring him that more emotional passion rather than more time would do the trick. After he did this he was told to close his eyes and imagine flying over the Earth, seeing it from on high. He was to add four puffs of wind, one in each geographical direction and say out loud each time: "The sea comes before the boat before the wind before the right direction is taken."

About eight months later, the family sent a newspaper article about how their son had convinced an old sailor to teach him how to rebuild a dilapidated sailboat. They accomplished it and the boy was now sailing on the local lake. More years passed, and we received a letter mentioning that he had gone to a state university and had become the youngest captain of the sailing team. Four years later, we heard he had graduated with a degree in geography, specializing in cartography. An internationally renowned cartographic society immediately hired him to make maps. We were sent a map he drew of the North Pole as seen from high above the ground.

Not only does a creative therapist throw raw meat, alligators, and pirates into a case, maps are made that reveal a wider horizon and alternative world. At the end of the creative therapy day, the therapist honors map making as long as it leads to unexpected treasure rather than the same old sinkholes and dead ends. You need more "meet" in your meetings with clients—meet them inside the circularly mapped world where the sea is ready to dissolve rather than solve or resolve their bitters and jitters.

14

HOW TO GET STARTED

Now that we are at the end, we can prescribe how to begin. Draw a circle exactly two feet in diameter on the corner of your therapy office's ceiling. Paint the sea and land, and then glue, tape, or thumbtack a cutout pirate boat. Make sure it has a pirate flag with these initials on it: *CTIP*. Never tell anyone that this is your secret pirate name for "Creative Therapist in Practice." When you need to see a flash of color or hear the wishes of the sea or the swishes of the sword, look in that direction and gently puff a bit of air. Wait for the creative wind to answer back and move you forward. It always does if you convince the other world that you are sincere and that you are ready to travel on the sea of change. One more thing, feel free to place a postcard or photograph of a New Orleans brass band in the other corner of your room, whether on the ceiling or the floor. Then you are all set to briefly turn your whole body in that direction and hear how the next note will make your performance more like jazz. We will be doing the same. Why sink when you can sing along to the tune of a bigger room?

APPENDIX

A 'Pataphysical History for the Future of Creative Therapy

Once upon a time in Vienna, before the fall of the monarchy, therapy clients would lie down on a couch and tell a story about their past to a new kind of wordsmith. The expert would then share a carefully construed interpretation to the client with the aim of giving deep meaning to the couch, hoping there would be less ouch in the client's life. This tailored alteration entailed a journey from the client's tale to the therapist's theoretical head and was thought to be therapeutic to the client and meaningful to the therapist, but not moving to the couch that never budged a single centimeter.

Many years later, at the Menninger Foundation located in Topeka, Kansas, one of the early bastions of psychoanalysis in the United States, Brad was employed with a job title he invented—"communications analyst." There he accidentally discovered that the psychoanalytic couch was given more attention than any outsider had previously noticed. The Menninger Foundation had a special carpentry shop where "analytic couches" were custom built to match the one in Freud's office, guaranteeing the correct angle for interpretation. However, the presumably bored Topeka carpenter was allowed to make one variation of the Viennese design. Two styles were offered to the analyst: one with a bookshelf at the end and another without, as if this choice unconsciously questioned where to situate interpretation—as the primary therapeutic action or as a secondary consideration that follows the body's action. And thus it was that a piece of furniture embodied therapy's choice of priority—to predominantly theoretically interpret or not. However, one aspect of the couch was not open to change. Analysts were strictly instructed to use "analytic napkins" to cover the headrest, with no other choice of material allowed. They were actually the same ones used by dentists, but no one except the newly arrived communications analyst asked whether both professionals made a living from utilizing an oral fixation and underscored the head while ignoring the rest of the body.

Back to Vienna: Freud and Jung had lunch in 1907 and hit it off because they talked for *thirteen* hours. That number thirteen must have jinxed them because they were like father and son until they took a journey to America two years later. On the ship, they analyzed each other's dreams and that didn't go well. Freud felt threatened and Jung felt insulted. That was the end of their dynamic interpreting affair. While each doctor continued to differentiate theoretical terms, the more important difference between the two practices was that the furniture changed. Jung gave up the couch and replaced it with a chair, believing that two chairs enabled the relationship between client and therapist to be more visibly recognized. However, interpretation continued to rule.

In this way, the furniture choice of either a couch or a heavy chair for interpretation-focused therapy was set for clients said to suffer from hysteria due to hidden, unruly plot lines. All this work with fantasy material inspired Sigmund Freud to declare a sexualized meaning for the social life of himself and everyone else in the world. This famous neurology rock star helped move sex from covert operation to openly discussed libidinal interpretation. More importantly, the *interpretation* of sex encouraged the elevation of mind's theoretical productions as the supreme protection against any live action inspired by the "dark inaccessible part of our personality … a chaos, a cauldron of seething excitations." (Freud, 1990, p. 91) In other words, Professor Freud suggested that interpretation reign over raw action, believing the latter too exciting for the interpreter's own good. While Jung was less worried about sexuality, he was equally worried about the chaotic intrusion of underlying energetic excitation so he, too, elevated the head to be lord over everything below.

Meanwhile across the Atlantic, F. Scott Fitzgerald announced the Jazz Age, which during the period between 1918–1928 brought flappers, hot jazz, and the roaring twenties. Though it was a time of prohibition, there was little inhibition. This is was the ideal time for the rebellious nature of America to launch its behaviorism. James Watson accordingly published *Psychology as the Behaviorist Views It* (sometimes called *The Behaviorist Manifesto*) in 1913. Pavlov and his Saint Petersburg dog act had won the Nobel Prize in 1904 (the first Russian to receive it) but its written work was not translated into English until 1927, the same year B. F. Skinner gave up his wish for a literary career and headed to Harvard to study psychology. There he exchanged his writing den for an operant conditioning chamber for pigeons that allowed no possibility of a text within the corridors and no visibility of the surrounding context that included Skinner's mind and body, his typewriter, and his own snacks.

Behaviorism spotlighted the countable action events found lying in a short behavioral sequence rather than the long speech uttered on either an elongated couch or a symbolic chair. Many years later during the advent of brief and strategic therapy, the behavioral action line was extended into an "interactional sequence" because more people's action was included. As the sequence was stretched, it was hoped that this new approach could further topple the decline of psychoanalysis and assume the top therapy position. All the behaviorists enamored by the unemotional observation of a sequence, short or long, found professional excitement in attacking any descendant of the interpreting cure. The equally removed and emotionally detached interpreter also induced personal arousal by the same hatred and attack, this time directed at both the non-interpreting behavioral sequencer and any competing interpreter.

The therapy tide historically and hysterically changed with B. F. Skinner's arrival in the same way it did later with Jay Haley in the 1970s and 1980s—they each had their brief moment of rewarded, reinforced, and socially triangulated fame when action was on the rise and interpretation on the demise. With the passage of time, their popularity would wane after being attacked and overthrown by interpreting antagonists who would explain that action or interaction alone drains away the privileged meaning of an interpreted life. The new interpreters of the late 1980s and thereafter were also unaware that in due time their victory would be reversed and cast aside by alternative action in the recycling of history's changing that enables the same future to rise and fall.

After the New York stock market crashed, people started asking "why" questions again and that was the end of naïve action-led success. Carl Rogers, another knight of interpretation, arrived to argue that the world and its fortune is what we conceive and perceive rather than what Skinner only measured pleasure to be. The Freudian slip and wedding gown continued to pass from one interpreting bride to another—Freud to Rogers to the narrative interpreters of family therapy and postmodern reflectors. The latter lacked the intellectual chops and writing skills of their European ancestors, so their moment of notoriety was more a brief footnote than a long-term theoretical foundation. In the other lineage, the behavioral tamers also passed on their reinforcement treats—Watson and Pavlov to Skinner, Watzlawick, Weakland, Fisch, and Haley to name a few who were instrumental in staying focused on the correction of an action sequence. Back and forth the fights have continued, disputing whether to highlight the action bits that are organized by sequence strips or the interpretive tidbits that provide a desired ideological fit. Again, what was missed by both lineages—their shared blind and deaf spot—was how behaviorists who wanted to throw away meaning offered professional action that was profoundly demeaning, while interpretative enthusiasts allergic to action-based influence partook in aggressive political action against their professional competition.

When it came to the furniture, most interpreters had moved from the lie-down couch to a sit-down chair. Both individual-focused behaviorists and systemic behaviorists working with interactional sequences involving several people sometimes added chairs or moved them around to enable observable performances of action. These different interior design schemes were inseparable from the theoretical debates that went on in spite of what anyone did or how any of it was interpreted, exactly like theology during the fifteenth and sixteenth centuries. Neither opposing side was aware of how they occupied the same room; only the furniture within it changed, and not significantly.

In the most enthusiastic days of family therapy (especially from the late 1960s until around 1985), a handful of pirate-like therapists mutinied and threw the furniture overboard, preferring to sail the whole family system into another kind of adventure. Many of these early pioneers regarded individual therapy as the absurd equivalent of only admitting one body part, like an arm or finger, into the medical doctor's office while the rest of the body was left outside. These "pure" family therapists insisted on working with the primary system of an individual's existential nexus. Some therapists would only see three generations and a few even rented auditoriums for whole social networks to be treated as part of the client system. Chairs were pushed back, making room for the family system to stand up, move around, and be re-sculpted, reorganized, and recalibrated. The shock seen and heard around that world was that *performed therapy with whole systems* was placed on center stage. This rebellion changed the nature and placement of the furniture—the couch and head napkin were completely gone and chairs were lighter in weight so they could be more easily moved around as families enacted live scenarios. It was the most exciting era of the helping professions because it was paradigmatically different from psychological therapies, but it disturbed those who lusted for the crown but didn't have the systemic acumen and interactional performance chops to compete.

Old habits of viewing and doing aren't easy to break and making the paradigmatic leap to be a maestro of change requires Olympian dedication and hard work. Hence, it wasn't long until everyone sat back down in their clinical chairs again and returned to the former quarrel. Like the old song line, "You say 'tomato,' I say 'tomahto'..." some schools of therapy claimed the sung difference indicated two competing interpretations whereas other schools with different tools said it involved different action. More than a few were so frustrated with it all that they turned away from the whole therapeutic performance to assess the brain, watch the client's eyes move back and forth, compare test scores, gaze at mirrors, edit imaginary texts, or investigate the ancestry of a metaphor.

Some attention-hungry and disgruntled audience members, soon to emerge as the next wardens of the talking head way, started throwing tomatoes and tomahtos at the stage where the old masters demonstrated change in action. This began around 1985 with Lynn Hoffman's paper that claimed cybernetics was too concerned with power and control. Wanting to appear ethical and humble rather than lackadaisical and manipulative she and others publicly confessed that while they had formerly failed their therapy performance audition, a new insight led them to positively connote this outcome as a sign of success. Accordingly, with sophistry and rhetorical misdirection they announced their corrective mission was to bring back interpretation as the main show, devalue the importance of therapeutic action, and negatively attack any master whose performance noticeably evoked change. Like Freud, they wanted their action and relational interaction to be barely perceptible. Instead of facing a couch, they looked into the reflecting mirror to avoid getting more involved with the ongoing performance. This new breed of interpreter was the opposite of the "great originals" who preceded them—their sessions were boring (they even bragged about this) as they rambled all over the place, completely lost in conversational space. In other words, they performed like a beginning trainee who was unsure what to do with clients. Rather than responsibly face the needed skill acquisition like any other student of a performance art, they were led to believe that they were already enacting the new kind of mastery that was defined as avoiding any form of master performance. In summary, the legitimization of incompetence as a higher competence enabled the next generation of therapists to stop aiming for change. The tragic paradox is that they spent as many years learning how to further interpret and justify their inactivity as therapy—doing so when they could have learned how to more effectively act.

The overthrow of family therapy's original lineages occurred during the ascent of the "me" generation—those born between 1946 and 1964, who were credited with a new rise in narcissism in the 1980s. The combination of self-interest, individualism, mirrors, and reflections brought back a focus on interpretation that, in turn, soon kicked out the family as the primary client system. The requirement that a whole relational system be included in therapy was dismissed, and if a couple or family showed up, they were regarded as a collection of individuals rather than as a whole system defined with a different class of metaphor. The verbal comments of each individual were taken as sufficient with no need to discern how experience, conduct, and even an individual's way of construing meaning are organized by patterns of interaction (which go unseen and unheard by untrained therapists).

Perhaps the most unethical political aspect of the new interpretation-focused therapists involved how they situated themselves in family therapy rather than individual therapy. They launched a bloody attack on strategic and action-oriented family therapists, doing so with a soft, meek voice, explaining that it was more therapeutic and polite to do as little as possible rather than be an unruly pirate on the ship of change that steers with a circular wheel. And so was squelched the ongoing dramaturgical revolution and its cybernetic form of systemic focus. "Systemic" and "cybernetics" were misappropriated and redefined to mean anything the interpreting author wished to indicate (which actually had always been an issue since the beginning of the family therapy field) so that soon the term had no practical or explanatory value. Adding the word "system" to virtually any metaphor made it systemic. Rather than work with family systems, therapists could now work with an interpreting system, a reflecting system, a conversational system, an endocrine system, a cortical system, or a political system. This was not the "system" the main pioneer family therapists had in mind when they differentiated themselves from individual-oriented psychotherapy. The overthrow of family therapy by non-family therapy orientations during the "me generation" threw the profession back to the former dualism that organized individual therapies. Once again, some therapists imposed their interpretations on clients while denying such action while others interpreted the action while denying they were doing any interpreting. Yet no matter how different their approaches, both kinds of therapists still performed in the same room and forgot that individuals live in a context whose systemic nature surpasses individual traits, experience, and expression.

The 1990s involved a heist of the family system—its politically calculated removal from the profession of family therapy was elegantly summarized and implicitly eulogized by Salvador Minuchin (1998) in his article, "Where Is the Family in Narrative Family Therapy?" Most clinics still had multiple chairs in the therapy room, but most of them were now empty. The field steered so out of control that eventually three of the main schools of family therapy programs (narrative therapy, postmodern therapy, and solution-focused therapy) had nothing to do with the founding premises of family therapy. There was no longer any system in so-called systemic therapy (H. Keeney & B. Keeney, 2012c). Even worse, family therapy organizations began investing their money in acquiring the legal right to medically diagnose, even though family therapy originally had rejected the notion that mental health resides in an individual's brain. By the turn of the twenty-first century, too many graduates of family therapy programs were already ignorant of their systemic ancestors and to this day perpetuate ideas and action that are antithetical to the fundamental premise of family therapy. This devolution of family therapy left it in the same context as its competing individual therapists and uncertain how to justify itself as a separate profession.

Psychotherapy began with some brilliant theoretical fantasies written by well-educated scholars concerning the interpretation of the unconscious. In the beginning, the profession moved from the couch to heavyweight chairs. Then the interpreting therapist found its foe—the action-oriented behaviorist who cared less about heady flights into abstract meaning. Chairs were moved or removed to better observe the ongoing action scene. The first one-way mirror showed up in the behaviorist's clinic. The founding behaviorists were also intellectually rigorous in their method and text production. And thus, the first two paradigms of therapy were born: interpretationism and behaviorism.

The popularity and appeal of both paradigms went back and forth over the years and each sprouted several offshoots and subcultures. The third paradigm to emerge was the kind of family therapy that had a bona fide family system on its stage. While its room sometimes became bigger with more moveable and even removable furniture, its mutiny was short lived and its revolution almost entirely squelched. Those who couldn't enact its means of change replaced it with interpretation and action models that were now dumbed down to make them marketable for the workshop business where new teachers launched a career by immediately teaching a reframed part of a previous orientation. The cost of this pedagogical reorganization was a serious dumbing down of therapy performance and the quality of its texts. All in all, the history of therapy has not been a straight line of evolution. It has been a repeating circle whose enactment and intellect have recently become more reduced and less transformative with each round. Under the spell of naïve workshop models, the seduction of mystifying metaphors from intellectual disciplines not understood, the political demand for socio-statistical evidence, and the economic reliance upon psychiatric diagnosis, the profession is well on its way to becoming overthrown by the pharmacological corporations that offer the briefest, most researched, and most profitable model of them all. The most prized piece of furniture in this world is not the couch, chair, or mirror but the medicine cabinet.

This story marks the whole circular history of therapy from its beginning to its end. Or does it? Aren't its recycled changes more of the same old replay in spite of an altered metaphor or two? Or is some action or interpretation missing from the previous account? What does 'pataphysics have to say about all this? And what is "'pataphysics"? A 'pataphysical history production is a way of making the point that any action description and interpretative explanation of therapy's history is primarily influenced by the historian's personal preference for bringing forth a desired future. Certain events are selected like furniture and then arranged to create a staged setup for hosting a chosen future. Every historian of therapy advances their own style of therapy and later claims that what preceded it was just a failed attempt at reaching the very summit upon which they now stand. History's miseries and victories are redefined, re-connoted, and re-arranged to serve the historian's future design choice while postured as a mirror image of what took place. Such a historical account leaves its readership fenced in a constructed frame whose aim is to place the historian as the center star of the reminted therapy universe.

What can loosen the encapsulating hold of a rigged history and enable a creative crew of pirates to escape its predetermined future and have another adventure on a bigger, unknown sea? Enter 'pataphysics: it arrives to provide a different performance stage, experiential planet, and change-worthy future that invite more creative play. 'Pataphysics is an impossible to define trope invented by the French playwright, Alfred Jarry in 1893. It offers a spoof that reveals the absurdity of interpretation while lampooning the veiled vanity, political profanity, and rhetorical insanity of its interpreter. While a 'pataphysical production seems to occasionally ring true, it's also felt to be equally absurd, though more creatively evocative than any feigned final word. Monsieur Jarry mandated that an apostrophe precede its spelling to help others know it was not just a pun. As much fun as this kind of play may be, it's dead serious when it comes to striking down any interpreter of the past, present, or future, now exposing them as trying to stake down a final claim for how to legitimize the performance of theater, science, art, therapy, or life.

Aaron Hillyer (2015) suggested that while the "metaphors" of grand-scale, socially accepted interpretations are one degree removed from consensual reality, the "'pataphors" of 'pataphysics are twice removed. 'Pataphysics arrives to lampoon and harpoon with humor, sharp insight, and fuzzy logic, breaking up whatever is regarded as an established and readily observed reality, especially for those in creative decay and incapable of play. 'Pataphysics does not bring another dimension or coloration to *the* world, but creates an immeasurable, unknowable atmosphere that seems not quite real, yet is far more fascinating than what is uncritically presumed to be real.

The leap into creative therapy involves not distance from the client, but separation from a "reality" whose exaggerated reifications and fantasy observations rely upon action that re-invent and recycle its incessant interpretations. This is not a map coming before the territory nor is it a new pair of spectacles that change the view of the world. It is neither more nor less than mapping, viewing, and even territory construction. Furthermore, it is equally not limited to replacing the sensory hegemony of the observed observing eye with audition, listening, dialogue, diatribe, hermeneutic construal, or social constructionism. It's something more capable of fluidic difference and this difference dynamic is impossible to indicate for it is an escape from finalizing indication in order to have another round that begins with evocation rather than representation. The creative therapist does not act in order to find meaning and does not need to understand the meaning of an action before enacting it. Confused? The 'pataphysicist celebrates confusion for it is the first sign of being liberated from a former reality and the preparation for taking a different kind of non-informed action.

Creative therapy, in the spirit of this version of a 'pataphysical history, outrageously proposes that there is something vital that has been missed in the previous histories of the debates, conflicts, and battles of therapy's back-and-forth, non-Hegelian, ping pong game between its legions of actors and squadrons of interpreters. The multi-sense kaleidoscope and anti-sense stethoscope of 'pataphysics reveals that all the fussing and cussing over all these years have been mostly about variant preferences for room furniture and its placement, while ignoring that the clinical room has remained the same. We are not just speaking of couches, chairs, windows, mirrors, paintings, Egyptian statuettes, books, and Persian rugs. The objectification of metaphors and constructs has led therapists to treating problems, solutions, people, culture, and the like as hard objects that are placed in the room like furniture. Freud placed his client on a couch while working on the deeply embedded story that floated out of the patient above the upholstery as if it were a book to edit and interpret. Fritz Perls placed the invisible inner parts of his clients into chairs and then talked to them as ghosts. Virgina Satir later preferred a "parts party" with the many parts of a person role played by other actors rather than have a gestalt one-on-one encounter. Problem finders and solution seekers made each of their nouns more real in order to justify the need of a therapy designed to handle them. Finally, narrative therapists capitalized "the problem" (now a "Problem") and placed that reified part in external space to have a political whack at it. In conclusion, disagreements over the choice and placement of furniture and accessory objects were extended to include relating to the categories of experience and people as additional furnishings.

The 'pataphysical history of family therapy similarly regards it as a family feud over room decoration—whether to include an observing team bench, conversational chairs, a couch, a bookshelf empty or full of theories, the number and kind of windows, white, purple, or multi-colored walls, a video camera, a telephone, and any other decoration. At first, "systemic" indicated the family's performed interaction in a room that was met with therapeutic intervening action rather than theoretical habits of interpretation. For example, family members were frequently asked to change their seating arrangement or directed to talk to one another instead of the therapist. Later, in the hands of former psychoanalysts from Milan, "systemic" was redefined as a type of interpretation given to the family at the end of the session. Here it seemed the whole family was lying on an oversized Freudian couch. For the action-oriented therapist, a one-way mirror enabled better strategic prescriptions to be constructed from behind the scene. For the interpreting therapist, action was avoided in favor of a back-room formulation of hypotheses that were turned into family interpretations. In the beginning, these interpretations were meant as the treatment action, but later were reinterpreted as sharing a reflection that didn't mean to suggest anything.

Creative therapy cares less about prefixed interior decorating and ignores the battle between whether to exclude the mind's thoughts or the body's action. It aims to existentially expand the room to welcome all kinds of creative expression that embodies the dynamic of change. Any furniture or decoration may be introduced as a prop that inspires a change-bound improvisation. It's the whole room's degree of expansion, creative thawing, and atmosphere of excitement that matter more than the furniture, whether it is made of wood, upholstery, metal, plastic, or linguistically hardened metaphors. Creative therapy offers this practical advice to feuding therapists: get over arguing what kind of furniture is involved and be very careful about turning extracted parts of human experience into hard objects—this tends to make everyone in the room more dissociated and as mad as a hatter, something that is only useful when guided by creative rather than ideological hands.

Make sure the room is big enough so it feels *both real and beyond real, enough to arouse curiosity but not enough to readily disqualify.* If it's too real, it will bore. If it seems unreal, it will not inspire exploratory action. Make it both physical and 'pataphysical, a breeding ground for imaginable and unimaginable change. Even forget about perpetuating the difference or relationship between knowing and action, interpretation and performance. Change the reality of reality to make more room for your being different. And then be different again in ways that set a creative transformative fire that spreads to others.

Creative therapy with all its wordplay and lively action is candid and upfront about its intent: *it invites therapists to get on the big stage of change and get on with the show*. When breaking a leg is advised, break open whatever holds back the human capacity to experience taming a shrew, entering a midsummer night's dream, getting over the fear of Virginia's Woolfe, welcoming a raisin in the sun, arranging a homecoming, and finding a way to exit and no longer wait for Godot. If needed, go ahead and hypnotically induce a purposeful amnesia for whatever was heard or taught about fearing the stage, snearing at the action, and demoralizing the desire to change. Take a thousand steps away from any toxic advice that paralyzes therapeutic performance. Interpretation is action and action cannot help but be interpreted in multiple ways, but the latter's presence or absence is more resourcefully steered by the ongoing changes of the performance rather than the evangelical imposition of an ideology.

Act on behalf of changing the stage, the play, and all actors involved. If not for you, do it for your clients who deserve more than a napkin for the head or a curtain that divides so a reflection, interpretation, or disengaged recommendation is all that is fed. Do it for your mother because she'd be happier if you took more action for yourself and others. And don't forget to do it for the healing ancestors whose dramatic action will be long remembered after their mumbling critics are forever forgotten along with their furniture disputes. Act in order to change, the only means of getting to know you and another. Would you rather secure the furniture or raise the curtain? Would you rather have a conversation or a transformation? This is the question whose broader range of answer is cracked open by simply taking the action that voices it while feeling the depth and breadth of the choice. Don't get lost in an archaeological dig for meaning when the absurdity of inventing a poetic ditty or witty one-liner and not explaining either is wiser than the literal claim that all is an interpretive exchange. Act to bring life back to therapy's performance. Change again in order to wake the muse who inspires how to act next.

The theater of creative therapy improvises in order to benefit from the differences and changes born in a changed performance. To know how, we must reenter our ongoing 'pataphysical, historical drama again. Do you know what it means to miss New Orleans? Jazz as a music form was born there around 1895. Here the rooms are outfitted with more than Victorian couches and chairs. Brass, reed, string, and rhythm instruments are placed on every stage. Music is in the air. Do you already miss Viennese pastry? There, art nouveau has arrived to introduce more natural curves, soon to shift into art deco, modernism, and all the other aesthetic experiments. 1895 was a pivotal year, the beginning of a lean toward all kinds of different futures. Sigmund Freud managed for the first time to analyze a dream. The "dream of Irma's injection" became the cornerstone of his *Interpretation of Dreams.* Freud immediately wrote a letter to Wilhelm Fliess, the man he admired and called "the Kepler of biology" who was a crackpot otolarynologist who operated on Freud's nasal membrane to cure his neurosis and then followed up with cocaine treatment. Freud wrote: "Do you suppose that some day a marble tablet will be placed on the house, inscribed with these words: 'In this house on July 24, 1895, the Secret of Dreams was revealed to Dr. Sigmund Freud.'"

This was the year that Carl Jung stopped going to church after many clashes with his theologically oriented father. In the same year, his father was diagnosed with cancer and died with Carl by his side. His father's death immediately liberated his persona and that year he transformed from being a reclusive "bookworm" to becoming an extroverted party animal who received the nickname, "The Barrel." Later he built a stone tower with his own hands. While Jung worked with stone, Freud collected mushrooms from the field. Both got their hands dirty outside of therapy and each found ancient relics in curio shops and stuffed them into their offices. Arguably more live action in the room would have better tilled the creative ground, encouraged further curiosity, and uncovered theoretically unexpected hidden treasure. In other words, less attention to stone and mush would have cleared more room for a performance surprise.

Zigzagging back to New Orleans and Basin Street: while Europeans were dreaming, collecting artifacts, and altering interpretations, Buddy Bolden was crowned the "King" of the cornet as his band played the first improvised music of jazz in dives, honkytonks, funerals, and brothels. We need not speculate on how the same furniture was found in the settings that staged both the origin of psychotherapy and jazz. Suffice it to say that an injection dream on a Viennese couch, a barrel amidst Basel's stones, and some horn-blown improvisation in a New Orleans parlor decorated with European furnishings brought us therapy and jazz.

Another forgotten fact is required for a surprise ending to our historical tale: in 1895, Oscar Hammerstein I opened the Olympia Theatre, a massive grey stone building that was inspired by French Renaissance design. It was a performance complex in New York City's Times Square district that included a theater, a music hall, a concert hall, and a roof garden. This was also the year that August and Louis Lumiere displayed their first moving picture in Paris. Other exciting developments in performance included new actors taking the stage: Grace Young became the first woman to receive a doctorate in Germany at a university built by King George II of Great Britain, who made sure to outfit it with a riding hall and fencing house where words were not that important. Simultaneously, W. E. B. Du Bois was the first African American to receive a Ph.D. from Harvard University, a place also influenced by Great Britain's higher educational and architectural design. Note that its founder, Reverend John Harvard, had a mother born in theatrical Stratford-upon-Avon and a grandfather who lived down the street from Shakespeare. However, John Harvard ended up being sculpted as sitting in a chair rather than standing on a stage, where he remains today in Harvard Yard presiding over a pile of sculpted books.

Equally important to the 'pataphysician, 1895 was the year that baseball giant Babe Ruth was also born of German ancestral parents in the Pigtown section of Baltimore. Few know that his father was a lightning rod salesman, an often-forgotten feature of any house. Also relevant, but sad to say, that across the ocean in County Tipperary, Ireland, Bridget Cleary was killed by her husband because he believed her to be a fairy changeling. A British drinking song was soon thereafter composed about the same place: "It's a Long Way to Tipperary." Interpreting therapists might be fascinated to know that this same place also became the home of "Coolmore Stud," the largest thoroughbred breeding operation in the world. While the British men were singing bar tunes and the Irish were breeding studs, forgotten was Bridget Cleary whose husband, on trial for her murder, argued that she had been abducted by fairies and replaced by a changeling—he had only destroyed the changeling. This is what led to the popular Irish nursery rhyme: "Are you a witch, or are you a fairy/Or are you the wife of Michael Cleary?" Nothing is known about the furniture in their house other than she had a recently acquired Singer sewing machine that likely did not make a singing tone.

While all this may make our history sound like a mystery or fairy tale, we don't want anyone to miss remembering that there is nothing like an Irish ghost to help a lost talker find the blarney stone. Nothing else can change the performed manner and skillful influence of talk. Ireland is where the ire and poetic fire may be found that awakens creative imagination and the uncommon action needed for change—including doing something in the opposite manner. Kissing the Blarney Stone while leaning backwards is a leaning action rather than another invented meaning. This is what magically precedes being able to charm with more clever talk. Therapy could use a bit more Irish ale to help prevent the performance ailments that come from getting intoxicated with tales.

Complexity science, fractals, and strings have taught the world that everything can be explained by the close relations of far, near, and in between. Therefore, the flapping of an Irish fairy's wings can be linked to a Calcutta breeze or associated with anything at all including a dreamt coffee at a Vienna café table or a frothy beer at a baseball bench in Yankee Stadium. Intoxicated with centuries of synchronicities and untold possibilities, the world was made hungry for the mythical, physical *swing* of Babe Ruth's mighty bat in the fifth inning of game three of the 1932 World Series. This strong swinging action, the cracking sound, and the crowd's thunderous applause were heard all around sports eternity. Babe Ruth, also born in the magical year of 1895, fulfilled his immortality by first pointing his finger toward the blue afternoon sky, suggesting he'd hit the ball far over the wall. In that particular inning of the game, held in Chicago's Wrigley Field, he pointed to a spot high above center field before the pitcher delivered the pitch. Then the world forever changed and would never be the same again: *Crack!* A sound never to be forgotten was made by his bat as the Babe, the Bambino, and the Sultan of Swat made direct contact with a spinning, stitched, leather ball. He drove that major league baseball 490 feet to the deepest part of center field, with some saying it went past the flagpole perhaps with the help of a breeze from Calcutta, the flapping wings of Irish storytelling, and a belly full of hot dogs, cake, coffee, and beer—all partaken in a stadium whose seating and objects suited the mood of it all.

The hidden furniture rather than the lost meaning of this story is that Franklin Delano Roosevelt was sitting in a wood box seat behind home plate. F. D. R. wanted to jump out of his seat and do something that mattered after that mighty swing. He had not yet been elected president nor reincarnated to later sing on the Broadway stage with Annie. But reporters noted that Roosevelt laughed as the Babe rounded the plates. His laugh made front-page news, but it was only briefly mentioned in the story making it easy to miss. That giggle is what gave him the oomph he needed to help lead a country out of a mighty depression. Nothing lifts depression like healing laughter, no matter its cause.

Our epic drama of metaphor and 'pataphor is not yet over. Before Babe took his mighty swing in 1932 something else preceded it that must never be forgotten, and this brings us back to the importance of jazz. In February of that same year, Duke Ellington recorded his composition, "It Don't Mean a Thing if It Ain't Got That Swing." It was composed by Ellington during intermissions at Chicago's Lincoln Tavern in the Morton Grove area, the same name as another Lincoln Tavern in Chicago that later became known as Billy Goat Tavern. It was in that bar that a long-lasting curse was put on Wrigley Field and the Chicago Cubs. Whereas the Billy Goat created a nasty jinx, Duke Ellington offered a pleasant charm with his new song and lyrics. In a paper read at the Eastern Division of the American Society of Aesthetics, Donald Keefer (1992), a professor of philosophy, later summarized the importance of this composition: "Duke Ellington's song, 'It don't mean a thing if it ain't got that swing,' can be read as a manifesto against the reigning intellectual culture of his time. Swing is emphatically about the body. Dionysian defiance of gravity. Whatever doesn't work its magic through the body doesn't count. There is a deep Socratic wisdom here: a life without swing, is not worth living."

A rare vintage photograph of Duke Ellington taking a swing of a baseball bat demonstrates his interest in both kinds of swing—jazz and baseball. As a child, Ellington was more interested in baseball than his music lessons. "President Roosevelt (Teddy) would come by on his horse sometimes, and stop and watch us play," already a sign that the other Roosevelt would later watch Babe Ruth's physical swing during the time when Ellington's musical swing was in the radio airwaves.

Our 'pataphysical juke joint point is that Duke Ellington's hit record surely excited the right kind of rhythm that inspired Babe Ruth's motion, resulting in a once-in-an-epoch swing and hit that, in turn, swung the mood for a soon-to-be president to turn life around. Let's not be overly suspicious or excessively doubtful about the possibilities associated with the complexity of multiple relations, invisibly intertwined interactions, and parallel outcomes, especially when it comes to the 'pataphysical. Also, be aware that in 1932, Sigismund Schlomo Freud wrote Albert Einstein (who had no middle name) a personal letter regarding the state of the world and cautioned, "little good comes of consulting a theoretician, aloof from worldly contact, on practical and urgent problems!" (as cited in Kaes, Jay, & Dimendberg, 1995, p. 33). This did not mean what it may seem to mean on the surface—he wasn't being critical of Einstein's lack of practical know-how; he was referring to his own inadequacy. Professor Freud's letter praised Professor Einstein's noble efforts to make a difference in comparison to his own feeble attempts, though without context this might not be readily apparent. Freud knew he was a theorist more than he was an effective agent of change and admitted that he could offer little that was good for the problems of the world. He failed to notice that perhaps the same was true of trying to help clients change through methods that solely emphasize an interpretive means. Worth mentioning is that Freud despised music: "with music, I am almost incapable of obtaining any pleasure." (in Gay, 1989, p. 523) Einstein, on the other hand, was the opposite: "I live my daydreams in music. I see my life in terms of music … I get most joy in life out of music." It doesn't take a rocket scientist or a psychoanalyst to conclude that Einstein had swing and Freud didn't.

In that same year, 1932, Carl Gustav Jung gave a lecture entitled, "The Psychology of Kundalini" in which he warned against anyone wanting "to activate the unconscious means to awaken the divine." He had accidentally awakened his own unconscious and wasn't sure what to do with it other than put it back to sleep with incessant interpretation that bored enough to cause a snore rather than activate the roar of change. Though he visited the United States several times, it is not known whether he ever saw a baseball game. However, his theoretical therapeutic view has been used to explain the mythical curing powers of homeruns hit by Babe Ruth:

> *Jung's belief was that heroic activities in the outer world are manifestations of the hero within us all. This inner hero, if aroused, can perform miracles as described in Don Schlossberg's* The Baseball Catalogue: *"Eleven-year-old John D. Sylvester of Essex Fells, N.J., was given 30 minutes to live by doctors after a severe attack of blood poisoning … Young John spent his remaining time listening to the World Series. That was the day Babe Ruth hit three home runs in one game. Amazingly, John began to recover. The* New York Times *reported that … the boy's father and the physicians attributed the recovery to messages of encouragement received from Ruth and other stars. When Ruth hit his three home runs, the boy's fever began to break and his recovery began."*
>
> (McMartin, 1984)

Milton H. Erickson, a tone deaf, dyslexic, color blind, and prodigious therapist when it came to accessing a client's unconscious and formulating a strategic action plan, also wrote a paper in 1932 that was entitled, "Possible Detrimental Effects of Experimental Hypnosis." It ended with a conclusion that wasn't what most would expect from the title, which was only a set up for a final surprise: "In summary, then, the literature offers little credible information concerning possible detrimental effects of experimental hypnosis, although replete with dogmatic and opinionated denunciations founded on outworn and untenable concepts of the phenomenon" (Erickson, 1980, p. 493). More importantly, he indirectly invited the world to ignore the conclusions and practical advice of Freud, Jung, and all the subsequent reincarnations of interpretation kings and reflective queens who were afraid to act in a session. He also knew how to therapeutically use rather than interpret baseball. For example, Erickson told a twelve-year-old bedwetter about the many physical actions involved in throwing a baseball. His detailed discussion of timing and muscle control was heard by the boy's unconscious, providing a resource that could be applied to other parts of the body. Nothing about the presenting issue was interpreted or even mentioned—no sneaky pee was externalized, no psychodynamic envisioned, and no social symbol explored. Erickson utilized some well-executed blarney and the more real than mythical baseball to help a young boy hit a home run, knocking his misplaced body expression out of the bed and into the bathroom where it belonged.

While Jung had ancient tchotchkes similar to those found in Freud's office, his workspace was tidier with stained glass windows that reflected his interest in religious symbolism. Milton Erickson was a collector of ironwood carvings carved by the Seri Indians of Mexico and had cactus plantings in the yard of his middle-class ranch home in Phoenix, Arizona. As Brad's interview with the man who sold the carvings to him mentioned, Erickson liked to hear about the shamans of the villages where they came from. He would take imaginary flights to these places while holding a carving of an eagle or another wooden creature. Erickson used his collected objects to seed and activate the unconscious rather than as a frame of reference from which to interpret. Erickson's office didn't exude the ancient vibe of a museum backroom artifact collection like the clinical quarters of Jung and Freud. But he made up for any lack of perceivable mojo with his bolo ties and familiar objects that became magical by the way he surprisingly interacted with them. All three men had interesting furniture and office accessories, but none had any musical swing, though Erickson could pitch a baseball game. The important difference between them was found in how they related to their objects—either evoking or interpreting experience.

We were more recently informed by a daydream that the homerun Babe hit finally landed in purgatory, hell, or heaven, we are not yet sure. In this uncertain place, Lynn Hoffman and Michael White sit side-by-side in distant balcony seats, far behind Anna Freud, Karen Horney, Carl Rogers, Dr. Joyce Brothers, and all the other more historically renowned therapy interpreters. Then suddenly out of the blue, cybernetician Heinz von Foerster is spotted running across a baseball field wearing lederhosen and an Alpine hat with a colorful feather attached to its side. He leaps high to catch the ball hit by Babe Ruth light years ago. Heinz laughs like Roosevelt once did and then uses sign language to say that he will provide no play-by-play commentary, not mentioning the self-reflexive paradox of his communication. Then Heinz tosses a curveball to Gregory Bateson who seems to have arrived out of nowhere and the whole audience is immediately struck by this action—noticing that the nonlinear trajectory is more circular than previously imagined. It's a sphere caught in the afterlife atmosphere.

Heinz steps onto the pitching mound and now offers his verbal pitch: "I am sorry I didn't make more clear that the shift from the *observed* system to the *observing* system *does not* entail moving from *observations* of the observed to *observations* of observing. I should have paid more attention to how you would mishear the difference I intended to convey and that this mistake would throw you back in time to the linear-shaped couch in Vienna.

I should have selected and arranged the furniture more carefully before I spoke. I also should have taught you the Viennese Waltz so that you could better experience how turning in a circle is what enables forward movement."

Out of nowhere Michel Foucault or someone pretending to be him arrives dressed as an umpire who is screaming, "I am going back to Earth to haunt all oration and narration that produces scatology. Even postmodernism is little more than the excrement of modernity. In other words, whatever you said yesterday, drop it today! Why didn't therapists remember the advice I personally followed: "'The main interest in life and work is to become someone else that you were not in the beginning.' This specifically means that a therapist should arrive at the next session being someone different who is ready to do something not done before!" Michel's office, by the way, had more books than the other therapists mentioned, but he had very few knick-knacks. While he could throw a mean spitball, he also loved the classical music of Bach and Mozart. He likely heard the notes in an altered state due to his extreme indulgence in "recreational drugs." Regarding his attraction to death and self-mutilation as an affirmation of life, he sought sadomasochistic activity. His early adult years embraced Freudian dream interpretation, which he thoroughly enjoyed doing until he later found other ways to express his fondness for interpretation while making a postmodern hit. Following a debate with Foucault, Noam Chomsky was stricken by his amorality and spoke like a batter beaned by a baseball pitcher: "He struck me as completely amoral, I'd never met anyone who was so totally amoral." As all of this was revealed to the crowd that had gathered, Freud and Jung were heard mumbling overhead. They surprisingly were in agreement, saying that anyone building a therapy based on Foucault's ideas reveals an anal preoccupation with eschatological means that are confused with scatological ends.

Comedian George Carlin, now an angel sent to change the scene, offers some comic relief to what Michel left behind as a most unpleasant topic. He offers a small collection of aphorisms about excrement to remind everyone that a lot of the wisdom in the world can be re-articulated through waste:

- Taoism: Shit happens.
- Confucianism: Confucius say, "Shit happens."
- Humberto Maturana: The observer who is in the observed says, "In the shitting is the happening of shit."
- Alcoholics Anonymous: Shit happens one day at a time.
- Problem-solving therapy: Shit is maintained by shitty solutions
- Solution-focused therapy: Miracles are the real shit.
- Narrative therapy: Externalize that turd and then protest against it.
- Postmodern therapy: Don't you dare do any shit!
- Gregory Bateson: It requires a difference that makes a difference in order to recycle shit.

- Carl Whitaker: Shit doesn't happen; shit IS.
- Milton Erickson: If you encounter shit, utilize it.

As Carlin's wings carry him away, Jacques Lacan arrives, another couch dweller who unlike Freud thought music was a supreme art. He adds an analytical reprise: "The characteristic of a human being is that—and this is very much in contrast with other animals—he doesn't know what to do with his shit. He is encumbered by his shit ... Civilization means shit, *cloaca maxima*." (in Sinnerbrink, 1992, p. 352). Before going on, Lacan is interrupted by the even more outspoken family therapy trio of Salvador Minuchin, Jay Haley, and Braulio Montalvo. Minuchin loved art and theater and told Brad that he once treated Charles Mingus in a New York City emergency room and had no clue what he should say. Mingus had swing and Minuchin had swagger but neither knew how to jam with the other. Haley was less aesthetically inclined, while Montalvo enjoyed the limelight less but was the unsung hero behind the other two.

This trio now offers their three uncommon cents, first with Minuchin speaking: "Beware the flying couch from Vienna that begs to visit therapy offices anywhere in the world, making its inhabitants vulnerable to catching an oral or anal fixation." Montalvo pipes in: "The return of Victorian therapeutic morality and modernity is what produces the postmodern excrement of interpretation. Hiding the actor's visible interactions, interpretation ad hominem only redresses an old fixation on a biological function." Haley is more blunt: "Whether fantasizing a cleanup of body poop or a soiled narrative, the strategic action that matters is eliminated in its appropriation by interpretation."

Heinz von Foerster, who grew up in his grandmother's beautifully furnished Viennese salon (not that far from Freud's more modest apartment) that was filled with intellectuals, radicals, artists, and musicians, is ready to turn a dispute into higher cybernetic action. He grabs hold of a microphone to make sure he is heard above the others and continues: "I made my own plea for a cleanup of cybernetics at the Biological Computer Laboratory. I said 'laboratory,' not 'lavatory' for those of you who are prone to mishearing me. I formerly asked for the transition from a noun to a verb when I suggested that we move away from "the observed" to the dynamic action of *observing*. Yesterday I met Milton Erickson at a heavenly café and heard how he helped that young boy with an unregulated bladder. This is a perfect example of what I wanted to convey. Erickson worked with the dynamics of bladder control rather than interpreting the bed wetting." Heinz, now audibly and visibly excited, continues: "The circular dynamic of perception is a pairing *and* a comparing—the sensory-motor action that invents objects as well as strongly objects when that is said to be all there is. No knowledge, perception, or any kind of sense can be separate from action. Nor is a single diagnosis made without the intervention that brings it about. My former young colleague, Gregory Bateson, whose home had more books and Balinese carvings than furniture, moved toward this empty Zen, but not empty-headed, direction when he tried to say that there are different map-territory relations involved in the business of knowing—all the maps are sometimes territories and all the territories also serve as maps. The *difference* between them generates an interaction that can recursively generate different orders of map-territory relations where each side constantly switches its role in the relationship. When Gregory tells a story, please don't take this to mean that 'the story' is the thing. In the action of performed telling is embodied the story's construction and the whole of its interactions, conveying what no extracted word or phrase can ever say. Turn around for Gregory is again standing and I will proceed to act in a manner that confirms he has something important to express that is more than what can be named or interpreted. Do not interpret Gregory; experience him."

Gregory takes a long pause, smiles, and speaks after all these years: "I shall only mention that neither you nor I can specify what need be heard. No story can escape the vulgar reduction of being named an interpretation unless the tale zigzags about, unable to be caught by either butterfly net or the Alice of Lewis Carroll who could never tell whether she was up or down. Suspended between what's real and unreal, a performance does not narrate nor prostrate; it stands ready to sing and not mean a thing other than keep you less conscious of the unconscious circle that connects to correct and bring home a difference." It's clear that death has been good for Bateson's performance for he is even more poetically expressive. He also holds over his heart the William Blake illustrations for the *Book of Job* that his father passed on to him. Still unable to paint or perform music, Bateson remains even more adamant that talk unaided by aesthetics is unable to convey wisdom. Gregory's voice has become more musically influenced, however, and when he said the word "difference" it was with a shift of tone he hadn't produced before. That's when the sky above and the sky below thundered together.

Sliding down a zigzag lightning bolt, MIT mathematician Norbert Wiener appears. As an earthling, Weiner's hobby was to repeatedly read the *Encyclopedia Britannica* from A to Z and it was said that no other human being came close to the breadth of knowledge he held other than polymath philosopher Gottfried Leibniz or Weiner's colleague at M.I.T., Warren McCulloch, who slides down the lightning bolt right after him. Weiner, whose office often hosted a curious machine or robot that had more unpredictability than many therapists, dares to articulate some practical wisdom that is aimed at people who make a living trying to help others: "Avoid reduction for this is only a seduction that brings a circular disruption." John Cage and other artists Weiner inspired in his lifetime lift up their instruments to demonstrate a standing ovation. Warren McCulloch, whose office had a standup desk that faced an aquarium so more movement and change would be in his experiential surroundings, follows with his own words, a new version of his old aphorism now tailored for therapists: "Don't bite my cybernetics, look where it is pointing." After these super-minds spoke, God sang. Using every language at the same time, God, already changed into a Goddess, sang again: "Don't interpret and inter-pretend; act differently and interdepend."

The clouds clear and as the observers start to depart, Carl Whitaker and Milton Erickson arrive on a horse named "Unconscious," with guitars by their side. Dressed as an Arizona cowboy and a Wisconsin dairy farmer they speak and take turns interspersing these words as the drama turns: "Our 'pataphysical history ends where it began with two buckaroos named Hillary and Brad who ignored all therapy sacred cows except the maverick performances of a few. Following a ride around the cybernetic merry-go-round, the performing arts, and faraway healing places, they came back to find themselves in act two of the formerly hidden performance room. There they chose to live in 'a home where the buffalo roam, where the deer and the antelope play; where seldom is heard a discouraging word and the skies are not cloudy all day.'" These last words were not spoken by either Milton or Carl, but sung by an invisible chorus comprised of performing artists, healers, and an odd assortment of cybernetic jesters, polymaths, and merry pranksters.

As all of us now step into the play, all that can be said is that the rest of the ending to this always changing 'pataphysically historical, hysterically hilarious musical variety show is now handed over to you. Creative therapy's final act and new beginning is in your hands. Come on over to the big ranch of change where the furniture is free to change or disappear as are those who sit, lie, or jump on it. Before the surprise ending arrives, let us together heartily sing with that former New Yorker and once-upon-a-time cowboy songwriter, Cole Porter (1945), tipping our hats and paying respect to iconoclast therapists of the past:

I want to ride to the ridge where the west commences
Gaze at the moon till I lose my senses
Can't look at hobbles and I can't stand fences
Don't fence me in

Creative therapy is more than a Wild West Show. It's also more than improvised jazz. It knows how to hit and pitch, using the right kind of swing and swagger to move it along. It aims to better specify and further advance the operations that invite the unconscious mind tripper, the transformative interactor, the inventive intervenor, the improvisation-inspired changer, and the creative performer to play on the vastest stage. We invite you to pay attention to whenever an unexpected occurrence ripples the water of the deep well. Act differently in order to wake up more of the operations of change. Lean backwards to kiss the blarney stone while making the flip that places intervention before knowledge of the outcome. Then whatever is done and said shall forever serve change, but only for the moment when it's useful for inspiring and guiding the next round up in an improvised creative therapy rodeo. The creative therapist's dramaturgical knowing and change-desired action ride together toward the jazz funeral's sunset that will soon burst into healing's celebrative renewal. The bodies of creative therapy never surrender to a talking head or trivial debates over furniture placement, doodads, and fossilized words, but are found embodying the prize of the next surprise.

Take a Bow

Please feel no need to spread the word that the profession of therapy never left act one of the theater of change. It has only had one false start after another. It never arrived in the room that cooks; all its schools only took a different kind of look while wondering whether to lie or sit and then have a fit over those who chose differently. Frustrated by the performance impotence of theoretical pretense, it kept having a tantrum like a toddler learning to walk. Although a few former pioneers took a momentary creative step or two beyond the clinician's carton of theoretical boxes, sustained presence wasn't achieved. They would too often fall back into cramped treatment quarters and get locked into their own habits of thought and action. Though more creatively alive than their peers, they barely explored the higher atmosphere of change.

Entry into act two goes further than the past and present walls of therapeutic containment. At the beginning of the middle is where the performing artist brings wider expressive action to the stage. As its expanded atmosphere swirls and whirls with exhilarating emotion, every trance starts dancing with change. More importantly, the rest of the body comes into play to overthrow the rule of a former talking head that demanded a couch or chair to avoid taking a stand. Later in the middle act appears the healer of old ready to be a healer for any time from ancient to present and future.

"Quiet, please." There is another surprise that has yet to be told: Whether performing artist or ecstatic healer, no matter the degree of creative heat, whatever is set in motion leads to an ending. This is an entry into the final act where one finds the way the session began—its circular end. While all is well that ends well, it's even better when the end leads to an altered new start in a bigger performance space with a wider range of expression. When the session begins, everything said and done is considered prescriptive, never descriptive nor explanatory unless the latter enables the action to be better hidden inside its Trojan horse in order to get it across the body-mind (action-knowing) divide. Later the action is more clearly noticed to be an injunction to change and finally in the end, the announced prescription is clearly the main show as all eyes and ears attend to its delivery.

The future of creative therapy invites an adventurous exploration into the untamed performance territory that is none other than the old stomping ground of healers. First is needed the know-how to make the room big enough for an expanded home-on-the-range performance. We ask Ouroboros and its Recursive Frame Analysis mapmaker to take a bow, for without them the room would more likely remain small. Second is required the ability to keep the transitioned act in play as it gives birth to the emotion and commotion that brings whole bodies onto the performance stage. This is where change cooks, enabling the formerly frozen state to creatively melt and pass through the transformational gate. We ask the performing arts and the healing traditions to take their bow. Though formerly forgotten, we now appreciate and yearn for how they can swing and rock themselves across each juncture. Third is the curtain call for the creation of prescription, the final act of every show. We ask the inventors of prescription to take their bow for all the recipes provided. The final act may bring the greatest surprise and secret of all: every session, as well as the profession's history, must end 'pataphysically and never quite fully know what this means. In other words, beyond all the words is the prescription for action that aims to escape any final word. Being both real and unreal and even creatively more, it helps propagate a renewed beginning of new existential worlds and galaxies that are now an extension of the creative stage.

After all these years of furniture rearrangement and theoretical derangement, it's time for a radically different assignment. We already gave it. Did you miss or mistake it for another? Here it is again: *you are the performer and offspring of Ouroborus, not the entanglement of Gordian's knot.* Stop trying to straighten out your therapy life. Begin and end by circling around your changes. Walk away from therapy in order to find how to be creatively therapeutic and unexplainably change-worthy. Otherwise you'll miss all the creative jazz, never ride the vastest range, nor have the rhythmic swing, vocal ring, and ecstatic zing to hit a session out of the ballpark. Until we meet and cook again, happy trails to you that keep on circling the campfire.

REFERENCES

Anderson, H. (1997). *Conversations, language, and possibilities: A postmodern approach to therapy*. New York, NY: Basic Books.

Akstein, D. (1992). *Un voyage à travers la transe* [A Journey Through Trance]. Paris, France: Editions Sand.

Barron, F., Montuori, A., & Barron, A. (1977). *Creators on creating: Awakening and cultivating the imaginative mind*. New York, NY: Jeremy P. Tarcher/Penguin.

Bateson, G. (2000). *Steps to an ecology of mind*. Chicago, IL: University of Chicago Press. Originally published 1972.

Berry, W. (1997). *The unsettling of America: agriculture and culture*, 3rd edn. San Francisco, CA: Sierra Club Books.

Connell, G., Mitten, T., & Bumberry, W. M. (1998). *Reshaping family relationships: The symbolic therapy of Carl Whitaker*. Philadelphia, PA: Bruner/Mazel.

Erickson, B. A. & Keeney, B. (Eds.). (2006). *Milton H. Erickson: An American healer*. Philadelphia, PA: Ringing Rocks Press.

Erickson, M. (1980). Possible detrimental effects of experimental hypnosis. In Ernest L. Rossi (Ed.). *The nature of hypnosis and suggestion: The collected papers of Milton H. Erickson on hypnosis, Volume 1* (493–497). New York, NY: Irvington Publishers.

von Foerster, H. (1987). Cybernetics. In S. C. Shapiro (Ed.). *Encyclopedia for artificial intelligence* (Vol. 1, 225–227). New York, NY: Wiley.

Freud, S. (1990). *New introductory lectures on psychoanalysis* (The standard edition). James Strachey (Ed.). New York, NY: W. W. Norton & Company.

Gandhi, M. K. (2008). *Autobiography: The story of my experiments with truth*. Middletown, RI: BN Publishing.

Gay, P. (Ed.). (1989). *The Freud reader*. New York, NY: W. W. Norton & Company.

Hillyer, A. (2013). *The disappearance of literature: Blanchot, Agamben, and the writers of no*. New York, NY: Bloomsbury Academic.

Hoffman, L. (1993). *Exchanging voices: A collaborative approach to family therapy*. London, UK: Karnac Books.

Kaes, A., Jay, M., & Dimendberg, E. (Eds.). (1995). *The Weimar Republic sourcebook.* Berkeley, CA: University of California Press.

Keefer, D. (1992). "If it ain't got that swing: Musical performance practices and the possibility of musical meaning," Paper delivered to the American Society for Aesthetics, Eastern Division Meeting, Bard College. Downloaded October 6, 2018 from https://faculty.risd.edu/dkeefer/swing.htm.

Keeney, B. (Ed.). (1999–2004). *Profiles of healing, 11 volumes.* Philadelphia, PA: Ringing Rocks Press.

Keeney, B. (2011). The flying drum: The mojo doctor's guide to creating magic in your life. New York, NY: Atria Books/Beyond Words.

The Keeneys. (2016). *Sacred ecstatics: The recipe for setting your soul on fire.* CreateSpace.

Keeney, B. & Keeney, H. (2015). *Way of the Bushman: Spiritual teachings and practices of the Kalahari Ju/'hoansi.* Rochester, VT.: Bear & Company.

Keeney, B., Lawson, K., & Roose, M. (2010). "The 'J' and 'A' rocks: Homework assignment for handling jealousy, anger, and impulsive responses," In Howard Rosenthal (Ed.). *Favorite counseling and therapy. Homework assignments* (209–212). New York, NY: Routledge.

Keeney, B. P. (1983). *Aesthetics of change.* New York, NY: Guilford Press.

Keeney, B. P. (1991). *Improvisational therapy: A practical guide for creative clinical strategies.* New York, NY: Guilford Press.

Keeney, B. P. (2009). *The creative therapist: The art of awakening a session.* New York, NY: Taylor & Francis.

Keeney, B. P. & Ross, J. M. (1985). *Mind in therapy: Constructing systemic family therapies.* New York, NY: Basic Books.

Keeney, B. P. & Silverstein, O. (1986). *The therapeutic voice of Olga Silverstein.* New York, NY: Guilford Press.

Keeney, H. & Keeney, B. (2012a). *Circular therapeutics: Giving therapy a healing heart.* Phoenix, AZ: Zeig, Tucker, and Theisen.

Keeney, H. & Keeney, B. (2012b). Externalización en la terapia narrativa: Un re-surgimiento modernista del exorcismo. *Psicoterapia y Familia*, Vol. 25, No. 1, pp. 34–49.

Keeney, H. & Keeney, B. (2012c). What is systemic about systemic therapy? Therapy models muddle embodied systemic practice. *Journal of Systemic Therapies*, Vol. 31, No. 1, pp. 22–37.

Keeney, H. & Keeney, B. (2013). *Creative therapeutic technique: Skills for the art of bringing forth change.* Phoenix, AZ: Zeig, Tucker, and Theisen.

Keeney, H., Keeney, B., & Chenail, R. (2015). *Recursive frame analysis: A qualitative research method for mapping change-oriented discourse.* Fort Lauderdale, FL: The Qualitative Report Books.

Luepnitz, D. (1992). Nothing in common but their first names: The case of Foucault and White, *Journal of Family Therapy*, Vol. 14, No. 3, pp. 281–284.

McMartin, J. (1984). A Jung man's game that appeals to all. *The Baseball Research Journal Archive.* Downloaded October 2, 2018 from http://research.sabr.org/journals/a-jung-mans-game-that-appeals-to-all.

Minuchin, S. (1998). Where is the family in narrative family therapy? *Journal of Marital and Family Therapy*, Vol. 24, No. 4, pp. 397–403.

Neill, J. R., & Kniskern, D. P. (Eds.) (1982). *From psyche to system: The evolving therapy of Carl Whitaker.* New York, NY: The Guilford Press.

Oliver, J. (2006). The myth of Thomas Szasz, *The New Atlantis*, Vol. 13, Summer, pp. 68–84.

Porter, C. (1945). *Don't fence me in*. New York, NY: Harms.

Price, D. (1998). Gregory Bateson and the OSS: World War II and Gregory Bateson's assessment of applied anthropology. *Human Organization*, Vol. 57, No. 4, pp. 379–384.

Sinnerbrink, R. (1992). *The cook, the thief, his wife and her lover*: A discourse on disgust. *Continuum*, Vol. 5, No. 2, pp. 352–365.

Spencer-Brown, G. (1969). *Laws of form*. London, UK: Allen & Unwin.

Whitaker, C. (1976). Hindrance of theory in clinical work. In P. Geurin (Ed.). *Family therapy: Theory and practice* (154–164). New York, NY: Gardner Press.

White, M., & Epston, D. (1990). *Narrative means to therapeutic ends*. New York, NY: W.W. Norton & Company.

Watson, J. B. (1913). Psychology as the behaviorist views it. *Psychological Review*, Vol. 20, No. 2, pp. 158–177.

Watzlawick, P., Weakland, J., & Fisch, R. (1974). *Change: Principles of problem formation and problem resolution*. New York, NY: W. W. Norton & Company.

For Product Safety Concerns and Information please contact our EU representative GPSR@taylorandfrancis.com
Taylor & Francis Verlag GmbH, Kaufingerstraße 24, 80331 München, Germany

www.ingramcontent.com/pod-product-compliance
Ingram Content Group UK Ltd.
Pitfield, Milton Keynes, MK11 3LW, UK
UKHW022203190926
475702UK00003B/179
* 9 7 8 0 3 6 7 0 7 8 0 7 2 *